Treading Water with God
Lessons in Love While Care Giving

Treading Water with God
Lessons in Love While Care Giving

Veronica Kelly Badowski

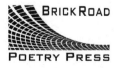

Copyright © 2013 by Veronica Kelly Badowski

Author's Note: All the Bible verses quoted in this book have been taken from *The Good News Translation*.

Scriptures and additional materials quoted are from the Good News Bible © 1994 published by the Bible Societies/HarperCollins Publishers Ltd UK, Good News Bible© American Bible Society 1966, 1971, 1976, 1992. Used with permission.

Cover photo credit: © Cammeraydave | Dreamstime.com

Library of Congress Control Number: 2012907720

ISBN-13: 978-0-9835304-4-2

Published by Brick Road Poetry Press
P. O. Box 751
Columbus, GA 31902-0751
www.brickroadpoetrypress.com

Brick Road logo by Dwight New

ALL RIGHTS RESERVED
Printed in the United States of America

For my parents
Martin F. Kelly, Florence Kelly Kiouttis, and George H. Kiouttis
who all loved me anyway.

My deepest thanks and appreciation to my husband Bill Badowski
and our loyal assistant who both made home care possible,
my son Keith Badowski who made this book possible,
my daughter Kelly Dawn Stokes, my Aunt Joanna Noble, Laurie Clyne and
our pastor Gloria McCanna who all cheered us on from the sidelines.

Introduction

As you read my story, you will find there are times when I was absolutely sure it was the right decision to care for my invalid elderly parents at home. It was during these times that I felt in tune with God's plan for my life, and I was learning the true meaning of the word *love*. It wasn't a flowery nice word used in a Mother or Father's Day card, but it came to mean giving up years of my time and energy to make sure my parents were happy and safe.

In the following pages, you will also read about the many days when I was down in a pit, lying flat on my face with no sunshine reaching me. This was when I did not want to take care of my parents anymore, and I thought I must have been crazy to think I ever could. These were the times I wanted someone else to take care of them because *I had enough!*

Of course, there was always the option of a nursing home. Two members of my family and a couple of friends have had to move loved ones into nursing homes. They visited them often and had an important part in overseeing their care. I do not criticize them for this decision, yet for me this never felt like the direction God wanted me to go.

My Heavenly Father gave gifts of love that made it possible for me to stay the course as my parents' caregiver rather than move in the other direction. My husband Bill and I had enough space in our house, so no one felt crowded. Bill was always willing to support and assist me in any way he could. My parents had money coming in each month, along with savings in the bank, so I was able to hire an assistant caregiver. God guided me to hire someone who was kind, compassionate, and loyal. Last but not least, God helped me every step of the way.

Before my parents came to live with us, they built their part of the house onto our three-bedroom ranch. It is beautiful with a separate entrance downstairs where there is a big all-purpose room. Up a flight of stairs, built to house a lift there is the kitchen with lots of cabinets and room for a table and chairs. There is also a big master bedroom with a full handicapped-bathroom nearby. Off the other side of the kitchen is one of our original bedrooms that we gave my parents to use as their television room. This part of the house is where eventually we put in two lift-chairs that were practical and comfortable for them.

When they moved in, I helped my mother with the curtains and the arrangement of the furniture. This kind of work seemed beyond my mother's capabilities at this point, but I didn't fully understand why until she began to show signs of premature dementia. Soon it was obvious to my stepfather George, my husband Bill, and I that we had a serious problem on our hands.

My mother was slowly descending into more and more confusion. She began to have extreme short-term memory loss and repeated the same stories over and over. Often she thought that I was two people and would ask me about the other lady. I'll never forget the day Mom asked me if I was her daughter. This question was not only shocking, but it was like a dagger in my heart.

As time passed, both my parents became more and more helpless. My mother came to the point where she spoke very little, did not know when she needed the bathroom, forgot how to walk, and could not eat unless someone spoon fed her. George, who was already legally blind when they first arrived at our house, made a slow, steady decline. At the end of his life, he had heart problems, needed kidney dialysis three times a week, and could barely breathe.

However, there were many good times together during the nine years my parents were with us. We often sat on the deck during the summer months and listened to the birds sing or enjoyed music from a local radio station. We went to church together, or we took an hour car trip to visit relatives. Even after we hired an assistant, my husband Bill and I tried to be home for every holiday, so my parents wouldn't be alone. I would cook extra big and fancy meals with the hope that the day felt special for them, as well as for us.

For the first few years, George and my mother were still relatively self-sufficient, but as time went on, they could do nothing for themselves. Sometimes the work I did as their caregiver seemed overwhelming. I was often tired, especially when our assistant had her weekly two days off. On those days, Bill would always help me, but I was still busy from morning till night. I would dole out pills, cook meals, feed my mother, cut up George's meals, cajole him to eat, supervise or give sponge baths, do general housework, take my mother to the bathroom, change her diapers, and be on guard that my stepfather didn't fall as he used his walker, sometimes recklessly. Often throughout the day, I found myself getting depressed. At eight PM, when George went to bed and took his last pills, I would say, *I'm going to fall asleep before you.* Then I would collapse into my own bed, unable to spend any time with Bill.

When our assistant came back, I was always happy to see her. Of course, it took me another day or two to fully recover, physically as well as emotionally.

Early on Bill and I learned that regular periods of rest and relaxation were a necessity. We would have burned-out way too soon if we didn't make time to do activities we enjoyed. Bill played racket ball, softball, and worked hours in his vegetable and flower garden. On days when our assistant was here or in between helping my parents, I prayed, took walks, and read inspirational books, or a suspenseful novel. Often I sat on the deck alone, enjoying Bill's potted flowers. I also found a little time for my hobbies: writing poetry, journaling, and making clay figures. Bill and I would attend church and also get away for short vacations, visiting our children and our grandson who live out of state. These activities kept my husband and I emotionally, mentally, and spiritually fit, so we were able to continue caring for my parents.

From the beginning, my hope was that this experience of care giving would help my soul to grow, making me a more mature Christian. I believe God's goal for each one of His children is to become like his own dear Son Jesus in thought and deed. However, way too often, I still found myself down in the dumps, feeling blue, because I was trapped by work and responsibility. Often I couldn't understand why God wanted me to continue taking care of my parents at home when it was so hard for me.

One day as I talked with a friend over the telephone, I came up with this analogy: *The job of caring for my parents feels like I have fallen off a boat, and I must tread water to stay alive. Only when I am safe and back on firm, dry land will I be able to say that I am glad I took care of them at home.*

After nine years of treading water, I finally made it to dry land. Both my parents are now in heaven. When I look back on all their physical problems, the pills, doctor visits, trips to the emergency room, car rides back and forth to the kidney dialysis center, visits to the wound care center, and hospital stays, I wonder how we all stayed sane. Yet God's guidance and love was always with us. I felt it strongly. He protected my parents especially when they were in the hospital. He provided Bill and me with what we needed to stay strong for each situation that came our way. If it wasn't for God watching over us, I doubt my husband and I would have been able to complete this huge job of caring for my parents at home. All praise goes to God, the Father, Son, and Holy Spirit.

*

As you read this book, you may want to chronicle your own experience as a caregiver. It doesn't matter what your journal looks like. It could be just loose pages kept it a folder or something more fancy. The important thing is to write about what happens and how you feel about it. As you write, don't worry whether your grammar or punctuation is correct. Unless you choose to share, no one else will see your work. Some days you might write only one word to express how you feel: *Peaceful. Tired. Angry.* The length of your entry has no bearing on its worth. Once you put a feeling or a thought on paper, you may want to ask yourself where it comes from. If the answer evades you today, maybe it will appear tomorrow or maybe weeks from now.

I have included sections called **YOUR JOURNAL**. If you choose to write about something else, these should be ignored. They are only there in case you need a jump off point on days when you can't think of anything else to put on paper.

Your journal will help you better understand yourself as a person and as a caregiver. Always remember you are human. *Only God is perfect.* When you begin to understand where negative feelings come from, I hope this will encourage you to be forgiving and gentle with yourself. When you are kind to yourself, you will have the energy to love others. This will in turn make you a better caregiver. Your job is a hard one, and sometimes the journey will seem way too long, but *with God's help you will succeed!*

Author's note: I am not a medical, psychological, or spiritual professional. Please check with your own professionals before making any decisions regarding your loved one's care.

For Now

A spider interrupts. She drops
from the apple tree, dangling.
I pinch the invisible string,
setting her on a plant.
Another one comes and falls near my feet.
She plays dead but eventually scurries away.

Now I continue to chronicle my life:
Repairs on the car cost
a preposterous amount.
One pill less makes Mom more alert,
but she still can't walk.
Stepfather recovers from heart failure
even though he's ready to die.
Our aging cat opts to sleep
rather than explore.
I suffocate, surrounded by oldness,
longing for playground days
with our grandson who lives far away.

A delivery interrupts. It's another
ominous scenario, wrapped in plain paper.
I drag it down into the cool dry cellar
and store it with the others on a dusty shelf.
I will open them, but not today.

For now I relax on a deckchair
where I absorb the warmth and
inhale smells of autumn olive
with tincture of potted jasmine
thrown in for fun.

Philippians 4:8

". . . fill your minds with those things that are good and that deserve praise: things that are true, noble, right, pure, lovely, and honorable."

Positive Thoughts

Both my parents were old and weak and needed my care in a multitude of ways. I had my husband's support and the help of a paid assistant, but the huge responsibility of watching over two elderly people weighed heavy on me. On this one particular day when George my stepfather was in the hospital, these were my thoughts: *I'm tired. I don't want to take care of my parents anymore.*

Every day I had been driving thirty minutes to the hospital and thirty minutes back home. While I visited with George, I had to be an alert advocate, making sure he got the best care. Then I would return home to my mother who was completely helpless with severe dementia. There was no escaping all my responsibilities.

I remember sitting in my car in the hospital-parking garage, longing for this commitment as caregiver to end. Then I felt as if God said to me, *stop thinking about it*. This was a simple, straightforward answer that actually worked. I stopped wishing for something that was obviously not going to happen anytime soon. When I switched my thoughts from despair to something pleasant, I felt relieved and at peace immediately.

It was just the right message at just the right time. This is why I am so certain that it came from God. He had reminded me of something that I already knew. For years I had been reading Dr. Norman Vincent Peale's books about faith in God along with positive thinking. I loved his books because they have never failed to lift my spirits. Now God was reminding me what I had learned, that I had the power to change how I felt by changing my thoughts.

*

Soon I discovered that the hard part was to prevent these negative thoughts from slowly creeping back. Often this would happen when I was physically and mentally tired. To prevent fatigue from setting in, I needed to make time for *play, rest, and prayer*. When I felt peaceful and rested, I had more energy, and it was easier to keep my thoughts *light and right*.

Instead of feeling sorry for myself, I had renewed faith that God gave me this work and was pleased that I loved and honored my parents by caring for them. Often I reminded myself that God was teaching me to be more like His own dear Son, my Lord and Savior Jesus.

YOUR JOURNAL

What are you thinking and feeling today?

TIP FOR CAREGIVER

Before my parents built an extension onto our house, and before we knew my parents would need it, my husband and I asked the architect to include a handicap-friendly bathroom in the blueprints. This meant the floor space had to be large enough for a wheelchair to enter and turn around easily. It also meant it had to be large enough to accommodate a roomy shower stall with a seat.

If you don't have a handicap bathroom for your loved one, there are still things that can be done to make the one you have safer. My husband added stainless steel handrails alongside the toilet for my stepfather who was unsteady on his feet. Also handrails can be mounted near the bathtub for safe entry and exit. There are also shower and tub chairs available. Look in the yellow pages for stores that specialize in products for the handicapped. It is amazing how many helpful things are out there.

Attitude Adjustment

There is a gloomy dragon, settling in my soul,
munching at the tender sprouts, straining to survive.
Sometimes the beast annoys me; I try to kick it out, but
there are days I give up, feeling sorry for myself.
Then God reminds me, my attitude is wrong.

Again I am reminded of the love and loyalty,
caring for elderly parents who must lean on me.
The sad dragon roars, but before I blink,
it turns pasty pale and begins to shrink.

God knew what I needed, a turn from sad to hope.
Now the flowers flourish deep inside my soul
where I choose acceptance of this sacrifice,
finding daily purpose for each day of my life.

I Thessalonians 5:16-18

"Be joyful always, pray at all times, be thankful in all circumstances. This is what God wants for you in your life in union with Christ Jesus."

The Power of Prayer

Only when I meet our Lord Jesus face to face will I understand how much good was accomplished every time I made time to pray during the years that I cared for my parents. Sometimes though I was so busy that prayer seemed to be just one more thing on my to-do-list. I knew this was the wrong attitude since prayer always brings me closer to my Heavenly Father. And when I draw near Him, He gladly shares with me His guidance and wisdom.

When I remained close to God, He gave me what I needed to continue as a caregiver. He gave me thoughts that kept me uplifted throughout the day, and He helped me to make the right decisions for my parents. Even though a part of me resisted at times, I realized it was essential that I prayed my way through this labor of love.

YOUR JOURNAL

What do you need help with today? When you pray, remember God will always provide what is best for you and your loved one.

TIP FOR CAREGIVER

Our assistant and I discovered that using an extension toilet seat saved our backs when we transferred my mother from wheelchair to toilet and vice versa. Also it was easier for George to sit and stand since his legs were weak.

A Walk with You

Let me talk with you, Lord.
I'm full of those complaints.
This work you've given me
saps all my strength.

First we'll speak of simple things,
the flowers, how they grow,
the cold winter snowflakes,
each different from the next,
and our pets that soothe us
when we are so stressed.

Next we'll talk
of wondrous things,
what the Father did.
In His own dear image,
He made the human race.
When we went astray,
He sent us You, His Son
to save us from our sins.

Lord, now please remind me
how much you sacrificed,
why the Spirit stays inside,
chiseling at my soul.

The more we are together,
I begin to understand.
You are just a prayer away,
because you are my friend.

James 1:12

"Happy are those who remain faithful under trials, because when they succeed in passing such a test, they will receive as their reward the life which God has promised to those who love him."

Ambivalence

While I took care of my parents at home a few people called me an angel. If they only knew the real me . . . *I'm no angel!* Often I gave my rebellious spirit too much energy by wishing I could pack my bags and run away from all my responsibilities. At best I was an angel only occasionally.

I tried to be good by picking up the gauntlet each day and deciding once again, *I can do this!* I tried to brush the negative thoughts away and continue to give my parents the tender loving care they deserved.

Sometimes I felt as if this was the way it was supposed to be, my parents living with Bill and me. Then other times, I felt like it was a mistake, and I wished they had never come. These opposing thoughts fought inside me so much that I thought I must be a bad person.

Then I'd remember what my Aunt Joanna told me when I telephoned her one day to complain.

You know what that means? You're human.

She was right. No person can give perfect love. Only Jesus our Lord and Savior accomplished this perfection while He was here on earth. Now it was only with the Holy Spirit's guidance that I kept trying to do the best for Mom and George.

YOUR JOURNAL

Write about a time when the words *you're only human* would have been exactly what you needed to hear. Remember, you can't be a perfect caregiver, but you can be a good one.

TIP FOR CAREGIVER

Since my mother could no longer follow instructions such as, *keep your eyes shut*, we used no-tear products when we shampooed her hair or washed her face. This made the job painless for all of us.

Ambivalence

God calls me to climb
a mountain.
One foot goes up while
the other goes down.

Ephesians 5:1-2

"Since you are God's dear children, you must try to be like him. Your life must be controlled by love, just as Christ loved us and gave his life for us as a sweet-smelling offering and sacrifice that pleases God."

Compassion

George's arms were full of bruises from everyday wear and tear. At ninety-five his skin was paper-thin, and he was on blood thinners, making the problem worse. Sometimes I felt sad, just looking at him. I would think to myself, p*oor George, he is so old and frail.*

I also felt deeply sorry for my mother who all her life was such a loving and caring person. Her brain had failed, and she wasn't herself anymore. A good thing she didn't fully comprehend the seriousness of her dementia. *Poor Mom.*

These extra intense emotions I had for my parents only lasted a few seconds here and there throughout the day. Good thing they were short lived; otherwise, I would have burned out with sadness. Although, wherever I found myself emotionally, I knew that my Father in Heaven wanted me to always be a kind and patient. My job was to help my parents have the best life possible under the circumstances.

Often I would wish I didn't have this job as caregiver. Some days were easier than others, but God was always nearby with His love, wisdom, and encouragement. He gave me everything I needed to continue being a caregiver, and His help was just a prayer away.

YOUR JOURNAL

Write about what the word *compassion* means to you as you care for your loved one.

TIP FOR CAREGIVER

Since my mother was incontinent and also prone to sores due to poor circulation, a nurse at the wound care center suggested that we use a special cream that protects against a breakdown of the skin. Your doctor or wound care specialist will be able to recommend the latest and best protective barrier for your loved one.

Winter Lookout

Outside there are
gray clouds,
gray grass,
gray weeds.
I shiver at the bare chill,
longing for the warmth of summer.

I need a hug from God.
Any little happiness will do.
You see, I have this pain,
not sharp but dull,
sapping away my joy.

I want my foot on the gas pedal till sunset
with nothing pressing back home.
Chocolate and pizza will do just fine
as fill for this sinkhole of mine
while my eyes become faucets
for sure, quick relief.

Of course,
what I really need is hands of the clock
in reverse,
ticking back shared memories
Mom misplaced along the way.

2 Chronicles 6:14

"He [Solomon] prayed, 'Lord God of Israel, in all heaven and earth there is no God like you. You keep your covenant with your people and show them your love when they live in wholehearted obedience to you.'"

God's Constant Guidance

While I worked as a caregiver, often I contemplated that this job was one of the greatest and most important things I have ever done for God. Being a good wife to my husband Bill and, with his help, raising our two children, Kelly and Keith, ranks up there as important work also. All these accomplishments were done with God's help and guidance.

Somehow though I felt so much more sacrifice was involved in overseeing my parents' care. Our children became less and less dependent as time went on. It was a joy to watch them grow and accomplish things like using the toilet, dressing, and feeding themselves. We were proud of them when they came home with good grades and joined worthwhile clubs and activities after school. With my parents, the process was in reverse, and each day brought them closer to total dependence on our assistant, Bill and me.

Since I believed God was pleased with me, as I made sure my parents were safe and well, I also trusted him to give me the wisdom and strength I needed each day. Often I allowed myself to complain and feel blue, but God was always there. He never failed to remind me that I had power over my thoughts. I could choose to be peaceful or discontented. He gave me the wisdom I needed to pick myself up and continue this commitment.

YOUR JOURNAL

Do you feel that God wants you to do something special for him by being a caregiver? It is my opinion that not everyone can be a caregiver, and God only calls those who are capable physically, mentally, and emotionally.

TIP FOR CAREGIVER

Sometimes my mother needed to be left on the toilet for as long as fifteen or twenty minutes. Since she could easily fall off the seat, our assistant or I would stay with her the whole time. When it was my turn, I would try to get other things done at the same time such as brushing her teeth, combing her hair, washing her face, and applying moisturizer to her feet and legs to prevent dry skin.

Now

The graceful monarch
makes her rounds among flowers.
Hours ago she was a gray lump
on the underside of a dark bush.
Now bathed in sunlight,
she is praised
for her beauty as she dines
on the best nectar.

When I embraced sacrifice,
my soul emerged
from its dark place.
Now illuminated with purpose,
I am called an angel who cares
for those who need me.

Proverbs 3:3-4

"Never let go of loyalty and faithfulness. Tie them around your neck; write them on your heart. If you do this, both God and people will be pleased with you."

Is It Worth It?

As I worked to keep my parents healthy, I often asked myself if it was worth all the effort. There were the endless doctor and emergency room visits, tests and hospital procedures, three days a week of kidney dialysis, physical therapy sessions, diaper changes, the ordering and organizing of medication, cooking healthy meals and so much more. Often I felt trapped and overwhelmed by the work and responsibility.

My mother had severe dementia and could not carry on a conversation any more. She used to make several sweaters every year, but now she thought a ball of yarn was something to eat. She and George used to go to church every Sunday and visit with friends often. Those days were over, but both of them still found moments of enjoyment.

Mom appeared to be peaceful and happy as she watched television, ate her meals, and listened to us talk. When we spoke to her directly, she made good eye contact and would often say a word or two. She also enjoyed rides in the car, watching the world go by. When we are at the doctor's office or a restaurant, she intently listened and watched everyone around her. I came to the conclusion all the work I did trying to keep her alive and well was worth it.

George still had his own mind, but didn't seem quite as content as my mother. He had been legally blind for quite some time, and now his kidneys had failed. This meant he had to have dialysis three times a week. He had to be jabbed with a huge needle in order to be hooked up to a machine that cleaned his blood for three and a half hours. Sometimes I thought my good care was just prolonging his agony.

Then I would remind myself that even though George's world had become small, he still loved breakfast, especially my oatmeal special that I made with nuts and non-fat eggs. He loved to listen to music on the radio as he sat outside on the deck. Also, he looked forward to the many evenings when I read to him from a book. I decided that my work caring for him was well worth it.

Yes, my parents had some quality of life left, but most importantly they were children of God. Their lives were sacred. In God's eyes, their lives had meaning and purpose. He placed them in my care and made it possible for Bill, our assistant, and me to continue doing this work. While they lived in our house, they felt secure, peaceful, and loved.

Only God knew exactly the right time for them to leave this earth. I didn't have to worry that somehow I had gotten in the way of this process. God was in control, not me. His wisdom and power was and continues to be above human understanding.

YOUR JOURNAL

Is there something you do each day that helps promote and preserve your loved one's quality of life? Remember, don't underestimate the power of a smile or hug.

TIP FOR CAREGIVER

During the cold winter months, I used an electric heater in the bathroom, so the room would be nice and warm before I brought my mother in there. When I changed my mother's diaper or dressed her, she was much calmer because she was not chilled.

For safety's sake, I removed the heater before the bathroom was actually in use. We all know that water and electricity don't mix, and backing into it could have easily burned someone.

Another Hospital Visit

I walk toward his room, and
the spur on my right foot grumbles,
we've been here
fourteen times this week.

His food tray has arrived,
but he's fast asleep.
I tap the toes of the man
who served
on a World War Two destroyer.

Ancient eyes open, but
he'd rather choose oblivion
over the plight of sinking metabolism.
Reluctantly his mouth opens
for mealy meatloaf and bland broccoli.

Later I encourage him,
your circulation needs stimulation.
Slowly he acquiesces.
He disembarks from bed,
steers his walker
across the room, and
sets anchor from a chair.
We speak of weather, world, and
those back home, but
too soon he launches himself
on course for his white berth.
He slides under cover, and
I kiss his oily head.

On the elevator, I question my service,
since he outlives his internal organs.
The door slides open, and
without a doubt, I will be back tomorrow.
With pail and mop in hand,

I will board the ship,
the one with the rusty engine below.
Once again I'll swab the deck
until it shines like new.

Hebrews 4:16

"Let us have confidence, then, and approach God's throne, where there is grace. There we will receive mercy and find grace to help us just when we need it."

The Blue Zone

I always had this feeling of impending doom just before our assistant had a day or two off, when I had to do everything for my parents from morning to night. Often I felt defeated before the day began. All I could think of was how much work I had to do and how exhausted I would become as the day progressed. *If only my parents could take care of their own personal needs,* I kept thinking.

Eventually they both needed assistance getting out of bed, washing up, dressing, taking their medications, eating, and moving from room to room. For me the worst job of all was putting my mother on the toilet and changing her diaper.

At some point, I would remind myself not to wish this commitment away, because, in reality, I was wishing my life away. There is a saying, *live each day as if it were your last.* To me this meant I had to find some joy and peace in little moments throughout each day. Certainly, there were things to smile and laugh about as I spent time with my parents. George had a good sense of humor that helped all of us feel better about his declining health. Then there was the natural world around me, such as the sunshine coming in the window or a hummingbird landing on Bill's flowers that grew on our deck. Joy was all around if I was open to it.

*

One morning I got up early, so I could read something inspirational before starting the day. I also did some praying. I felt more positive and determined to have a good day now that I had taken this time with the Lord.

Today, I would kid around with George, trying to keep him in an upbeat mood. My goal would be patience and gentleness as I took my mother to the bathroom, washed her, and fed her, remembering all the while, how much she loved me all these years. I would take pride in making a delicious meal for all of us and keeping the place neat and clean. Last but not least, I would happily help Bill in any way I could.

Even though I had a full day ahead of me, I would make time for a few minutes of rest. I would sit outside, watch the birds, and soak up the sunshine while my parents took a nap. If it rained, I would work on my hobby of writing poems or reading. All the while, I would look for peace, joy, and delight with God's help. He would give me the wisdom and guidance I needed to get through all the many everyday chores.

YOUR JOURNAL

How will you prepare your mind and heart each morning for the day ahead?

TIP FOR CAREGIVER

My stepfather was legally blind and also had developed weak legs, but each day he would sponge bathe, shave, and brush his teeth with just a little assistance. I helped him disrobe, except for his underwear, and then he sat in the wheelchair lined with his terrycloth robe. I pushed the wheelchair in front of the bathroom sink where everything he needed was within easy reach. Before leaving, I soaped his washcloth and gave him a couple of other wet washcloths for rinsing purposes. Since he locked the wheels on his chair before he stood up, my hope was that with the sink in front and wheelchair in back he would stay standing. If his legs gave out on him, hopefully he would collapse back into his chair. It was a bit risky, but I felt that preservation of his independence was that important.

Even though I closed the bathroom door for his privacy, I tried to stay within earshot. Later on things did change, and I needed to be in there with him, but for a long time it made him feel good that he could still handle his own personal care.

The Blue Zone

In case you've never been here,
I'll show you all around.
It's below the basement
in a bunker underground.
The place is poorly lit,
and there's nowhere to go.
The only game you play here
is called Sourdough.
This is how it's done, and
there's no other way.
Declare you are defeated
at the start of each new day.

All complaints are gloomy,
and also extra loud,
all shoulders sag
with heads deeply bowed.
The winner's plight is worse
than all those down here.
The loser still has hope,
so he can't shed a tear.
The prize is a deed
to a sad, lonely space
where joy is not a word, and
nothing good takes place.

Then without delay
the loser must get out.
There was never ever
one little, single doubt—
the Blue Zone is home
to those who want despair
while others need happy thoughts

as much as they need air.
The title of a winner
you may want to choose,
but as for me, my friend,
I would rather lose.

Colossians 3:13

"Be tolerant with one another and forgive one another whenever any of you has a complaint against someone else. You must forgive one another just as the Lord has forgiven you."

Only God is Perfect

Often I had to remind myself that only God is perfect. Occasionally I forgot to give my mother her second calcium pill or the pill that regulates her blood pressure. One evening Bill and I put my mother to bed without turning on the alternating air mattress. This meant she spent the whole night on the deflated, bumpy mattress. A couple of times, I forgot to put George's nitro patch on, which regulates blood pressure. Once when I filled his weekly pill organizer, I forgot the Synthroid that allowed his body to metabolize food. It wasn't until several days later that I noticed my mistake. When he had shingles and didn't feel well enough to eat, I forgot to give him a supplement drink before he went to bed.

The list goes on and on of things I have failed to do. It's amazing that both my parents were never harmed by my forgetfulness. I thank God for keeping them safe.

Even our professional assistant forgot things that she knew were important. At first I was angry, but then I reminded myself, it was not fair for me to demand perfection when I was so imperfect. *Only God is perfect*, I told myself for the one-millionth time.

There was so much to remember such as pills, eye drops, nitro patch, hand washing, eyeglass cleaning, checking for bed sores, and under-the-breast irritations, etc., etc. Every day the list seemed to get longer and longer, much too long to keep it all in our heads, so I typed out a list. I made several copies that I kept on the counter in my parent's kitchen. As our assistant or I finished a job, we marked it off. Even with the list in front of us, we still forgot important things, only not as often.

If God wanted me to forgive others their imperfections, he certainly wanted me to forgive myself as well. This thought helped me feel more at peace every time I found myself simply being human as I took care of my parents.

YOUR JOURNAL

Think of something you forgot to do that you felt was important. Are there some steps you can take will help you remember next time?

TIP FOR CAREGIVER

Since my stepfather was blind and tired easily, there was always liquid soap in a pump available on the bathroom sink. Liquid soap is quicker and easier to use, and anything that could conserve his energy was definitely worthwhile.

Out of Sync

I watch from our deck
as nature runs on automatic.
The sun comes up on time,
hummingbirds siphon nectar,
butterflies circle each other, and
a robin peruses the blades of grass . . .

while I am consistently inconsistent.
Sometimes I don't elevate his swollen arm,
give her medication when due,
or get him ready for dialysis on time.

Internal turbulence capsizes me
into clutter and disorganization.
I am out of sync with myself,
and the God who made me.

I John 3:18

"My children, our love should not be just words and talk; it must be true love, which shows itself in action."

Sacrifice Times Two

It was hard for me to ignore the sacrifice my husband and I made as we took care of my parents. Our dream for retirement was to spend our summers in Maine, living near our daughter Kelly, our son-in-law Kurt, and our only grandchild John. Since our daughter is a teacher with her summers off, we would have had fun going to the beach with her and John. We also would have enjoyed watching our grandson playing Little League softball. Winters we wanted to live in Alabama near our son Keith and our daughter-in-law Christi. It goes without saying how much we wanted to escape the long cold spells of the northeast. These were good dreams, but now they were on hold because my parents needed us.

When the snow piled up in our driveway, Bill and I both agreed that we could easily do without the white stuff. He used a snow blower and a shovel as he cleaned the driveway, the stoop and stairs in front, and the deck and stairs in back. Often it took him about two hours to complete this monumental task. At least one mountain of snow always became high enough and lasted long enough to deserve a flag and a name.

Bill and I both agreed that for now we had to stay here in New York State and put up with winter. It would have been too hard for George to get used to a new dialysis center and a new kidney doctor. His steady decline had been steep, and his health was too fragile for him to be moved easily.

*

This is what love is all about, I realized, *being willing to make sacrifices for others.* My mother gave me her time and energy as she raised me, and later she became a wonderful mother-in-law and grandmother, always ready to help us in any way she could. George gave his time and energy as a kind stepfather, a good husband, and a supportive grandfather. They both knew how to give love, so now it was our turn to help them.

Also, it made me feel good to obey my Heavenly Father by accepting this sacrifice. All the help He was providing made me certain that it was His will I continue this work. It was God's blessing that our assistant was loyal and kind to my parents. Also it was a blessing that I had a caring husband who drove George to dialysis three days a week and assisted me when it was my turn to take care of my mother. Of course, Bill's help was the reason my parents were still home rather than in a nursing home. I thanked God for him.

I reminded myself that things aren't so bad. While Bill and I waited for our freedom, we lived in our mother-daughter house where the four of us had everything we needed to be safe and comfortable. We also had good friends and family nearby cheering us on from the sidelines.

YOUR JOURNAL

When you hear or read the word sacrifice, what goes through your mind? Is it a negative or positive word for you?

TIP FOR CAREGIVER

In my parents' bathroom, there was always a box of latex or vinyl gloves on hand. They were invaluable for protecting our hands when we had to wipe bottoms, applying cream medications, and cleanup messy spills. Also the gloves were a big help when our assistant and I moved extremely soiled laundry from the hamper to the washing machine.

Worse Things

Tests confirm a problem
with the cat's heart.
She is still the same,
begging for fresh water in a mug,
jumping on her favorite bed,
rolling on her back when
we use friendly tones—

the way I speak to my mother
when I bring her to the bathroom,
change her clothes,
comb her graying hair.

There are worse things
than caring for an aging parent.
I am still the same:
sleeping next to my husband,
waking to the smell of coffee,
eating warm, sweet oatmeal.

Psalm 103:13-18

"As a father is kind to his children,
    so the Lord is kind to those who honor him.
He knows what we are made of;
    he remembers that we are dust.

As for us, our life is like grass.
We grow and flourish like a wild flower;
    then the wind blows on it, and it is gone—
    no one sees it again.
But for those who honor the Lord, his love lasts forever,
    and his goodness endures for all generations
of those who are true to his covenant
    and who faithfully obey his commands."

Following My Heart's Desire

Often I thought about a future when I would have time to do all the things I couldn't squeeze into my life as caregiver. At some point, I asked myself, *is this really true, that I don't have time now?* I decided to take closer inventory of my schedule.

Sure, I was busy: I had full charge of my parents two days a week from morning until they went to sleep in the evening. On a regular basis, I ordered their medication, did their banking, and took them to doctor and dentist appointments, not to mention the housework on both sides of the house and preparation of meals for the four of us. Even though the work seemed endless, there had to be a way I could carve out some time for myself each week.

It was tricky, and some days it didn't work at all, but with a bit of organization, I made time here and there for things that were important and fun for me. Usually early in the morning or when my parents napped on the days I took care of them, I would make time to write in my journal, exercise, compose poetry, and do some crafts. Everyone needs some downtime for their mental health, and I was no exception. When I did my hobbies, I felt more positive and happier inside.

God had known what I would need before He gave me this job. I couldn't possibly have done all the work alone, so He provided me with a husband who helped me every step of the way and an assistant who was dedicated to my parents. Even with their help, it was still up to me to give myself the gift of time.

YOUR JOURNAL

What are some activities that you have put on hold because you don't think you have the time? Are there moments here and there, when you do have a few minutes for yourself? Remember, everyone needs to have some fun, unwind, and rest in order to stay mentally, physically, and spiritually healthy.

TIP FOR CAREGIVER

I always tried to keep an extra supply of toilet paper in the bathroom to save steps later. It also was a big help to my legally blind stepfather when I put a new roll in the holder, not allowing the almost finished one to run out when he was in there.

Patches of Joy

I take a break,
walking in the neighborhood.
Occasionally the sun plays
hide-and-seek with clouds,
reminding me it's still there.

Today my life will imitate nature.
While I do housework,
dole out pills, make meals, and
feed my mother with a spoon,
dark dread will slide in and out
somewhere between my neck
and bellybutton.

Ahead the field
of goldenrod brightens, and
the sun warms my face again.
I know patches of joy will
come and go
while I work in God's plan.

Proverbs 8:12

"I am Wisdom, and I have insight;
    I have knowledge and sound judgment."

Evolution

I will always remember the wisdom of my late Aunt Joanna's admonition: *If she takes good care of your mother, don't worry about the housework.* My aunt was referring to our assistant.

I'll admit I was extremely disappointed, when our assistant announced she could not keep up with all the housework on the mother side of our house. She explained that my mother and George now required much more of her care and attention. It took me some time to feel at peace about this, but it helped when my aunt reminded me what was really important.

Slowly I began to overlook my original expectations of our assistant's duties. I came to appreciate and was thankful for her medical wisdom, her common sense in the face of a crisis, and her gentle kindness to Mom and George. Also she was extremely flexible about staying round-the-clock for several days in a row when Bill and I went to visit our son in Alabama or our daughter in Maine. Bill and I were greatly blessed to have her help.

Often I would remind myself that this was not the greatest job in the world, and if our assistant became tired and burnt out, it would not be a good thing. Then Bill and I would need to find someone else who might not be as kind, caring, and honest. Soon I began to think of our assistant as the sister that I always wanted. I was sure we would continue to be friends long after my parents were gone. Praise God that He sent her into our lives.

YOUR JOURNAL

If you were writing a list of responsibilities for your assistant, what would be your number one priority?

TIP FOR CAREGIVER

Baby wipes were wonderful for cleaning my mother's bottom whenever our assistant or I had to change her diaper. A combination of toilet paper and baby wipes often did the trick. Of course there were times when a nice warm soapy washcloth was necessary. Then there were those times when only a shower would do.

Ode to Our Assistant Caregiver

I'm sorry when I ride you, or
when I decide to chide you.
Of course no one is perfect.
It's wrong to disrespect
since I am flawed myself.

Hopefully there will be a day
when we both can say
my motives run crystal clear.

No longer will I be your boss,
no longer trapped in this crisscross
between friend and taskmaster.

Proverbs 17:22

"Being cheerful keeps you healthy. It is slow death to be gloomy all the time."

Ups and Downs

Sadness became a regular visitor in my soul as my parents' dependence grew. On the days our assistant was off duty, I was always down because there was so much work to do. I had to put one foot in front of the other and keep going. I knew that caring for my parents in a loving and gentle way was my purpose in life. Right now, it was God's will for me and my parents, but there were still times when I was tired, sad, and discouraged.

Often I wished that I could run away from home and my responsibilities. This negative mood seemed to have a life of its own, lasting a few minutes, a few hours, or even a few days. To be honest with myself, deep down I knew it was really me who was in control. The blues lasted as long as I chose to wallow in self-pity by thinking, *poor me; I have too much work and responsibility. I can't do this anymore. I don't want to do this anymore.*

Eventually, I would get sick of these unproductive, energy-sapping thoughts. Then once again I would remind myself that stay-at-home fathers and mothers care for their families. CEO's run their companies. Elected officials run our country. My job right now was to be a good wife to my husband and take care of my parents.

It was my belief that since God gave me this work as caregiver, He would give me everything that I needed to continue this commitment. For me prayer, uplifting Christian books, choosing to think positive thoughts, and a mild antidepressant, prescribed by my family doctor, were all helpful ingredients I used to fight off the blues. I was sure God was happy and pleased when I was able to care for my parents with a gentle, kind, and respectful spirit without feeling sorry for myself.

I always kept it in the back of my mind that if I lost my ability to climb out of the blues, I'd seek help. First I would pray for guidance. Then I would call my medical doctor or my pastor, asking for the name of a mental health professional. After some quality counseling and perhaps taking a stronger, more effective antidepressant, I'd be back to normal soon.

YOUR JOURNAL

Write about the last time you felt blue? Do you know why you felt this way?

TIP FOR CAREGIVER

When my mother's skin was still in good condition, we bought a quality protective barrier cream in large economical tubs and used it liberally on her bottom after showers and after some diaper changes. Your doctor will be able to direct you to the best product out there.

Sometimes They Sing

Out on the deck,
we bathe in bright sunshine,
Mom in her wheelchair,
George with his walker, and me
who feels one hundred and three.

The sky is clear;
the breeze blows cool,
no birdsongs fill the air.
Mom might be warm;
she might be cold.
I change my mind, but
still don't know.

I bring him water and
his hearing aide,
then tweak the radio.
Now the birds begin to sing.

Wish I were like birds up in trees.
Sometimes they fly in the breeze.
Sometimes they stay and sing.

Genesis 1:20-21

"Then God commanded, 'Let the water be filled with many kinds of living beings, and let the air be filled with birds.' So God created the great sea monsters, all kinds of creatures that live in the water, and all kinds of birds. And God was pleased with what he saw."

Nature's Peace

When I look out the window or go outside for some fresh air during the warmer months, I always feel happy and more peaceful. The birds, the trees, the flowers, and the bees all move and live as God planned from the very beginning. They are not hurried, confused, or overworked. If man doesn't get in the way of the natural world, all is as it should be.

When I was a caregiver, a walk anytime of the day was the way I recharged my batteries, but my goal was to get out early in the morning. The sun on my face, the fresh air, and a nearby bubbling brook filled my heart with joy and peace. This was one way I took good care of myself.

YOUR JOURNAL

Describe something enjoyable that you saw or heard the last time you were outside. As you visualize God's creation, you will find a few moments of needed peace and relaxation.

TIP FOR CAREGIVER

I discovered that pop-up wipes designed for cleaning bathrooms were helpful. They saved lots of time since no rinse was needed. Of course, for bigger more messy jobs I brought out the liquid cleaner, sponge, and mop.

Suddenly

I rescue my mother from a wet bed,
make her breakfast,
wash her hands, and
suddenly the sun is out.
From the glass slider, I watch
the brittle ice stuck on the apple tree,
melting it into droplets,
falling as sequins to the grass below
where warmth brings freedom.

I cannot mirror His love
as purely as droplets reflect the sun.
Nor can I be as compliant as melting ice
or as uncaring about my freedom.

I absorb the scene outside, and
hard, cold fear softens.
The shiny branches
make me thankful as if I were seeing
the buds of spring,
peeking out their tender heads.

I John 4:7

"Dear friends, let us love one another, because love comes from God. Whoever loves is a child of God and knows God."

A Good Man

My stepfather George came into my life when I was eighteen, and I never had a close relationship with him. He married my mother two years after my father passed away from an aggressive form of lung cancer. At the time, I was just beginning to experience life outside high school, but I still needed my mother. She and I were always best friends, and perhaps I was a bit jealous, not wanting anyone to come between us.

Even though I knew George wasn't trying to replace my father, I still resented his presence and tried to avoid being in the same room with him as much as possible. I couldn't understand how my mother could marry him, but on an intellectual level, I knew I should not feel this way. Certainly someday soon, I would move away, and I didn't want my mother to be alone.

Fast-forward more than thirty years and here I was taking care of George and my mother in earnest from the time they moved into our house and my mother's mind began to fail.

Still George was not one of my favorite people, but now we had a history together. For many years, he helped Bill and me in whatever way he could. Often he would drive our children to and from school functions and later from their jobs. I remember fondly how he took me to a road test when I accidentally allowed my license to expire. Also, he came with me on long-distance rides to a doctor's appointment. He was good company, and the trip was much more pleasant with him in the car.

When my mother's mind reached a point where she needed more care than I could handle alone, George resented the fact that I had to spend their money for an assistant. His resentment was extremely upsetting to me because I didn't really have a choice. If I wanted to keep my mother out of a nursing home, I needed help taking care of her.

Eventually, George made a complete turnaround. Often he would say, *if it wasn't for you I'd be dead already. I don't know what would happen to your mother and me without you. God bless you. I love you,* he would say to me just before going to sleep. My feelings for him definitely warmed and grew during the years I took care of him.

Of course, my love for George was always different then the love I had for my own father. Despite that I will always appreciate his kindness to my family and me. I am thankful that he was good to my mother, putting security and fun back into her life. All God's children deserve help and respect, but George made it easy to take care of him because he was a kind, good man. Perhaps I actually came to love him during the nine years he and my mom lived with us.

*

It became important to our assistant and me that George was content in his last years of life. Little things meant a whole lot to him such as his recliner placed near a sunny window, his favorite TV shows tuned in, and food that tasted good even without salt. Being there to talk with him and help him get dressed was also important to him. After that he looked forward to evenings when I read out loud, usually from a Robert B. Parker book. It became clear to me that I couldn't be happy unless I knew things were okay with George.

Now that he is gone, I miss the times we shared a book, and I miss our heart to heart talks. He was a good listener, but more importantly he was a good man.

YOUR JOURNAL

Have your feelings for your loved one changed over time? If so, in what way?

TIP FOR CAREGIVER

When days passed without Mom having a BM, we never gave up trying to solve her problem. We knew this was serious, even life-threatening. We called the gastroenterologist often, not allowing him to give up either. Eventually, he ordered the right combination of procedures and medication that solved her problem.

Bedtime Story

When the sky is no longer lit,
I'm tired, I must admit.
I go to the back of our house
where he waits with Mom his spouse
who is already snug in her bed, but
he stays up until I've read.

It's a mystery, plain and simple,
about a PI with just one dimple.
He wisecracks and then must fight.
Amazing he's still all right.
I read until my salvia dries
or lids lower on step dad's eyes,

but if we are close to the end,
of course we will extend.
Somehow we both stay awake,
and I read without a break.
When it's finished, we feel fine.
Our man solved the case in time.

Proverbs 2:3-6

"Yes, beg for knowledge; plead for insight. Look for it as hard as you would for silver or some hidden treasure. If you do, you will know what it means to fear the Lord and you will succeed in learning about God. It is the Lord who gives wisdom; from him come knowledge and understanding."

Daydreams

Both Bill and I looked forward to moving south where winters are shorter and milder than those in the northeast, where we would not need a snow shovel and blower. Our dream was to buy a house in Alabama near our son Keith and his wife Christi. In the summer when the south is hot and humid, we would head for Maine where our daughter Kelly, her husband Kurt, and our only grandson John live. There we would live in a trailer at a campground. It would be so very nice, seeing our children and our grandson more often.

This pleasant daydream ran through my mind often, but Bill and I could not make it happen since we did not want to move while my parents were still with us. George got to the point that he needed oxygen often, and he was prone to congestive heart failure. Just the trip alone might too stressful for his frail body. It would be hard for him to get used to new doctors and a new dialysis facility. It would also be extremely difficult, if not impossible, to replace our wonderfully flexible assistant. She was a gift from God that we did not want to give up.

Perhaps someday God would guide us to make these daydreams a reality. For the time being, I had to be patient and at peace with my job as caregiver to my parents. Each day, as well as our future, is always in God's hands, and I believe that His timing is always best.

YOUR JOURNAL

Is there a dream that you have had to put on hold until you fulfill your commitment as caregiver? How do you feel about this?

TIP FOR CAREGIVER

When it became necessary, we rented standard and portable oxygen machines for George and hospital beds for both my parents. After we had forms filled out by the doctors, Medicare paid for each rental. The rental vendors provide these forms.

On the advice of the wound care center, my mother's bed included an alternating air mattress. Also, we were given advice by the doctors for the best angle position of my parent's head and feet, helping them breathe better and relieving pressure on my mother's wound.

Winter Thoughts

I look through the glass slider,
thinking of my friends
from the South,
wishing I were with them.

Here icicles hang
from the air conditioner, and
wind chills threaten
to make me a recluse.

At least the snow
is lovely in the sun,
sparkling like glittered felt
rolled out across lawns and houses.

And those pines are handsome
in their glazed overcoats
as they waltz
with Alberta Clipper.

Yet I long for a walk
with my friends
in temperatures suggesting a sweatshirt
where I don't become the ice sculpture
for a banquet at the bird feeder.

Lamentations 3:21-24

"Yet hope returns when I remember this one thing:

The Lord's unfailing love and mercy still continue,
    Fresh as the morning, as sure as the sunrise.
    The Lord is all I have, and so in him I put my hope."

Yet Another Pep Talk

When tragedy struck our family, I learned a huge lesson that helped me as I took care of my parents. Beth my son's first wife of seven years died quite suddenly in her seventh month of pregnancy. All of us were grief-stricken. Bill and I worried about our son's mental health. Would he survive this horrible blow?

Praise God, Keith continued to be strong and kept a positive outlook. He missed Beth immensely, and he was sad at the loss of their unborn child, but early on our son made an important decision. He decided not to be miserable. He believed God was with him and eventually happiness would come back in his life. Bill and I were proud of him and amazed at his strength in the face of tragedy.

While I took care of my parents, I also had to make this same decision; would I be miserable or at peace? On this one particular day, I was definitely sad, and I felt sorry for myself. The weather forecast promised 9-10 inches of snow; this meant our assistant would go home early. I would be the one to take my mother to the bathroom, wash her, change her diaper, feed her, and get her ready for bed. There were also many ways I had to assist George before he went to bed. On this day, life had not given me what I wanted, but it was in my power to gracefully accept things the way they were.

Once again, I would show my love for my parents by carefully attending to their needs. I told myself, *I'm good at this. God is pleased.* Also I would take a few minutes to do something fun and relaxing in between caring for them. Now I was ready to have a good day.

YOUR JOURNAL

What will be your choice today? Will you be miserable or at peace?

TIP FOR CAREGIVER

The room where my parents slept is the sunniest and warmest place in our house. In the winter months, they enjoyed the comfort of their bedroom during the day. With the help of my husband, we took out one of their bureaus and replaced it with a small couch. We put the back of the couch along the big window, so anyone who sat there would feel the warmth of the sun. Even when it was below zero outside, my stepfather could still enjoy hours in the sun.

Just Like Them

Outside it's too cold
for my elderly couple.
They don't see him blow
the white stuff into a mountain
while I build snow people
just like them.

The man wears a red necktie,
The lady a red hat.
He works the jokes.
She wins the friends.

Evenings they dance to Sinatra;
days they play penny poker;
after church they visit friends.

Soon a little rain here,
a little sun there, and
they're gone.
Next winter I'll build
another couple,
but once my parents are gone,
God won't create
another two just like them.

Ephesians 6:10-18

"Finally, build up your strength in union with the Lord and by means of his mighty power. Put on all the armor that God gives you, so that you will be able to stand up against the Devil's evil tricks. For we are not fighting against human beings but against the wicked spiritual forces in the heavenly world, the rulers, authorities, and cosmic powers of this dark age. So put on God's armor now! Then when the evil day comes, you will be able to resist the enemy's attacks; and after fighting to the end, you will still hold your ground.

So stand ready, with truth as a belt tight around your waist, with righteousness as your breastplate, and as your shoes the readiness to announce the Good News of peace. At all times carry faith as a shield; for with it you will be able to put out all the burning arrows shot by the Evil One. And accept salvation as a helmet, and the word of God as the sword which the Spirit gives you. Do all this in prayer, asking for God's help. Pray on every occasion, as the Spirit leads. For this reason keep alert and never give up; pray always for all God's people."

Lessons from Experience

On this one particular morning, I did not pray or read anything from my inspirational books which was usually how I started off my day. All I had accomplished was to roll out of bed, reluctantly. This morning like so many, many mornings before, I dwelled on the negative. I was tired of being a caregiver for two people who were becoming older and more dependent by the minute.

In spite of these negative thoughts I still believed that God would make it possible for me to continue this commitment. I also reminded myself that soon Bill and I would take a much needed short vacation in Maine since one of God's blessings was our assistant's willingness to stay with my parents for a few days.

It was unusual for me to be this down and blue just before a trip, but this particular morning I had allowed my mind to jump far ahead, thinking about how hard it always was to return to heavy responsibility after a short respite. I was already depressed about coming back home when I hadn't even gone yet.

If it were easy to give up caring for my parents, I would, but of course it was not. They were both old and frail. If I walked away from this commitment, they would have to go to a nursing home. Even if I visited every day to make sure they were all right, I knew they would not get that one-on-one attention that they got at home. George would feel displaced and lonely. My mother's sores might worsen without diligent care. Also, I would find it difficult to give up control and allow strangers to make important decisions for my parents. Here I was back to the same belief that I have had for such a long time now: God wanted me to keep my parents at home with me.

A few years earlier, my husband had to make a hard decision when his mother became seriously ill. With her in agreement, he decided on a nursing home that was said to be one of the best in New York State. He went to the facility a couple times a week to visit with her and to make sure she was all right.

However, when her condition worsened, the nursing home's doctor didn't seem to sense the same urgency that Bill did. A specialist was finally called, but three weeks later, he still had not come. My mother-in-law became so weak that we took her to the ER ourselves. By this time, she had pneumonia, and it was already too late. A few days later, she died.

It can be argued that it was my mother-in-law's time to be with our Lord anyway, but Bill felt his hands had been tied, preventing him from getting her the appropriate medical attention when she needed it. He counted on the wisdom of the doctor and nurses at the facility, but somehow they had been unaware that his mother had become gravely ill. This experience motivated him to cheer me on as we both took care of my parents at home.

From a purely selfish point of view, I often thought it would be nice just to visit my parents and then come home where I was not reminded of old age and impending death all the time. Instead I continued to put one foot in front of the other and relied on God to keep me going.

*

I understood back then and now that some people for various reasons must choose nursing homes for their loved ones. In my humble opinion, sometimes this is the only answer for families who do not have the benefit of enough space or do not have the money to hire an assistant. However, this does not mean that they abandon their loved ones. It does mean that now they must be alert advocates, visiting often, and making sure that their loved ones are getting the best care possible.

YOUR JOURNAL

Do you feel God is guiding you to watch over your loved one at home or at a nursing home?

TIP FOR CAREGIVER

After lunch our assistant or I transferred my mother from her lift-chair into her wheel chair. After a trip to the bathroom, we placed her in bed on her side. We decided to do this when the staff at the wound care center explained that off-loading is the best way to prevent bedsores. Rotating Mom's position often helped increase blood circulation to each part of her body. This after lunch ritual gave my mother the benefit of off-loading, and hopefully she also enjoyed the change of scenery.

His Wisdom

Lord, I don't want this work you've given me.
I feel trapped with no end I can clearly see.
I feel defeated and wish I were free.
It's hard to be needed and wonder, why me?
Your answer came as sure as my heartbeat.
Don't feel sorry for yourself; stop thinking defeat.

Psalm 103: 1-5

"Praise the Lord, my soul!
  All my being, praise his holy name!
Praise the Lord, my soul,
  and do not forget how kind he is.
He forgives all my sins
  and heals all my diseases.
He keeps me from the grave
  and blesses me with love and mercy.
He fills my life with good things,
  so that I stay young and strong like an eagle."

Carry On

After we had to hire an assistant, two days of every week I still had full charge of my parents' care. There was an endless list of things that had to be done: bring Mom back and forth to the toilet, wash her, change her diapers, dress her in fresh clothing, spoon-feed her all three meals, make sure she drank six cups of fluid, brush her teeth, and give her medication. Also I spent time sitting with her in front of the television, so she would not feel alone.

My stepfather also had become quite weak and helpless which meant I had to assist him as he dressed and make sure he didn't fall on his way to the living room or the bathroom. Then there was a never-ending battle, trying to get him to eat enough to keep his strength up while at the same time, restricting his fluid intake. Sometimes he just did not want to cooperate. By eleven AM, I was already exhausted with the rest of the day still ahead of me.

No wonder these days brought me the most stress and sadness. At some point, I began to ponder whether it was illogical to expect an overabundance of joy and happiness any day, now that I was caring for my parents. After all, life had not given me what I wanted.

Our children and grandson lived too far away for Bill and me to see them often. My parents were declining right before my eyes. George was frail, weak, and struggled to catch his breath when he walked just a few steps. Mom's dementia had progressed to the stage where she rarely fed herself and probably didn't know who I was. Last but not least, I missed the mother who had been my best friend all my life.

With all that had happened, it was amazing that I still enjoyed some moments along the way. It was God's blessing that we had an assistant who made it possible for Bill and me to get in some time away from care giving. I prayed, read inspirational books, and visited with supportive friends. Bill worked in his garden and played softball. Together we shopped, went the movies, and ate out. The blues would come and go, but God's wisdom and guidance continued to encourage me to pick up the gauntlet every day and carry on no matter how I felt about it.

YOUR JOURNAL

Is there one activity or hobby that your loved one enjoyed at one time that you can help them do now?

TIP FOR CAREGIVER

My mother watched TV all the time, and George liked to listen to it, so it seemed logical to us that they should also have one in their bedroom where they spent so much of their time. In order to save space, Bill installed strong brackets to hold the television up on the wall. Mom was able to watch it from her bed. Since George was legally blind, we didn't need to position the television screen toward him.

Driving on Blueberry Mountain

It can't concentrate
while trees flush red and yellow
as they twist in the breeze.
Fall is splendid this year
with no brittle brown, but

there is no way for me to prepare
for the cold melancholy ahead.
The robins have already fled,
and soon the branches will be bare
against an inconsolable sky.

Some things are inevitable
like the loss of my mother
before her death.
She still smiles,
but her words are jumbled
along with her memories.
Nowadays
I'm in no hurry to get home
where someone kind sits with her.

I stop the car and get out
at the edge of the forest
where I collect leaves
under a maple tree.
Back home I will stiffen them,
glue a pin on the back, and
sell them at the church fair.
Mom used to knit hats and gloves.
Back then they went like hot cakes, but
there was no warning of the end
before her time.
I stop picking and

gaze deep into the shadows.
Again I stumble into senseless longing,
but prickly bushes block my path.
There's nowhere else to go, so
I get back in the car and drive home.

Psalm 86:11-13a

"Teach me, Lord, what you want me to do,
 and I will obey you faithfully;
 teach me to serve you with complete devotion.
I will praise you with all my heart, O Lord my God;
 I will proclaim your greatness forever.
How great is your constant love for me!"

Second Thoughts

When Yaya, my Mom's mother, was still alive, our family would get together on Greek Orthodox Easter rather than the American one. We decided to go Greek once again and invited my mother's sister, Connie, and my cousin, Leah, and her husband Bill. Ever since my mother was in a wheelchair, it was easier for us to invite our family here for holidays. My Aunt Connie was also in nineties, just like my parents, but she was still able to walk and get in and out of cars on her own power.

Bill and I went to church in the morning which meant when we got home, I had last minute straightening to do. Adding further strain, I also insisted on making dyed eggs while our dinner cooked in the crock-pot. Somehow it all worked, and we sat down to eat at two pm.

At some point during the day, our assistant told me that George said his legs felt numb. Sometimes he didn't describe his ailments properly, so I wasn't sure he really meant what he had said. I wondered if his old hip injury was acting up due to the recent damp weather. Perhaps if I wasn't so distracted with dinner and visiting relatives, I would have taken his compliant more seriously, but for the moment, I didn't give it much thought.

Later our assistant said that George theorized he had a stroke because he had experienced double-vision. Now I was concerned. I kneeled in front of him as he sat in a chair. I asked him, *Are you all right?* He assured me that he was fine.

Now I know that I should have reacted immediately, calling the doctor and bringing him to the emergency room, but instead I told myself he wasn't in any immediate danger. After all, he did say he was all right, and I had been told that mini-strokes were common occurrences among the elderly.

It wasn't until the next morning after discussing these symptoms with our assistant that I felt the need to call his kidney doctor who was overseeing all of George's medical issues. I told the lady at the office that I didn't know whether there was any point in bringing George for testing since he seemed normal. I also told her that I was willing to bring him to the hospital if this is what the doctor wanted.

After I got off the phone, I contemplated other options. I knew George's heart doctor would immediately increase his blood thinner to prevent another stroke. I hesitated to go that route, because George had so many bleeding problems at dialysis when he had been on a stronger blood thinner.

At that time, the kidney doctor told us that dialysis patients usually don't have stroke problems. The heart doctor, on the other hand, remained convinced that George needed a larger dose. Back then George and I decided to listen to the kidney doctor instead. Now I was having second thoughts.

It would have been awful if a stroke only half killed him by paralyzing him. Perhaps it was time for George and me to side with the heart specialist again as to the level of blood thinner needed. Maybe I needed to act quickly before George had a major stroke.

YOUR JOURNAL

What is your plan when your loved one complains about something that you're not sure is serious?

TIP FOR CAREGIVER

George always wanted a glass of water on the night table by his bed, and we gave my mother her morning coffee in the same room. This meant we would often place drinks on their very old but lovely deep mahogany furniture. In order to protect these surfaces from spills, I covered them with clear plastic and decorative plastic placemats. This also brought some cheerful color in the room.

Nightlight Prayer

God bless you, he says
after I turn on oxygen for his sleep apnea.
He tells me God will listen to one so old.
Heaven knows I need a blessing.

Mom might not understand
but I say, *God bless you,* to both
before I leave their room.

They don't know I come back later
to pray in the glow of the nightlight.
Father, don't let them suffer.
Please take them fast and clean.

Ecclesiastes 2:26a

"God gives wisdom, knowledge, and happiness to those who please him . . ."

The Decision

Since a fear that George might become paralyzed by a stroke was strong in my thoughts, I called his heart doctor. After all, he was the one who warned us what might happen if George took a lower dose of blood thinner.

The triage nurse at the Heart Center said that George should go to the ER. While I knew she was right, I wished we didn't have to go there. Anytime I brought my parents to the ER, it seemed like we waited forever for a doctor, for tests to be given, and then the results of these tests. If after hours passed Mom or George were admitted, it would take another hour or more before a bed was available. In spite of that I knew a trip to the ER would be the fastest way for George to see a doctor and receive the increased medication that would hopefully prevent a serious stroke.

Since I notified George's kidney doctor that we were on our way to the ER, he met us there. Again, he explained the downside of too much blood thinner. It would be difficult to stop the bleeding at dialysis, and if George fell, it could be serious. I passed this information onto George, but in the end, my stepfather was willing to take the risk in the hope of preventing a stroke that might cause paralysis or death.

I felt thankful that God gave George and me the guidance and wisdom to make this hard decision. Praise God! He does come through with answers even when we don't know we need them.

YOUR JOURNAL

Are there ways you can be more organized if you arrange your loved ones clothes, food, and toiletries to maximize your time and efficiency?

TIP FOR CAREGIVER

My mother's clothes hung on the right side of their closet; George's hung on the left. Toward the middle were the clothes they wore most often. As the seasons changed, I would dig out what they needed and put it toward the middle. This made it easier and faster to find everything in the morning when there was so much to do anyway.

God's Wisdom

There is no drought with God's wisdom.
It is dependable as night and day.
When we ask for it,
the rain pours, the sun shines, and
it arrives like tomatoes in the garden
when a hundred ripen all at once.

Psalm 119:76

"Let your constant love comfort me,
    as you have promised me, your servant."

Mistakes

Hospital mistakes and infections are in the news constantly, and every time George or Mom was in the hospital, our assistant and I were alert advocates. We did not take anything for granted. By expecting the worse, we were in a position to stop a mistake before it happened or at the very least correct it in a hurry. I often joked with George saying, *They tried, but they didn't kill you this time.*

This time my stepfather was admitted to the hospital with a possible mini-stroke, resulting in no permanent damage. I thanked God for this. His kidney doctor reluctantly put him on a stronger blood thinner in order to prevent another stroke.

All seemed well, but I suspected George's usual regimen of medication would somehow get mixed-up while he was there; it always did, especially the two different eye drops for his glaucoma. George was legally blind from macular degeneration, but he still had minimal vision at the corner of his eyes. It was imperative that he took medication to preserve what little sight he had left. This time the nurse assured me they would be able to get these medications right away. Not trusting this to happen, I left his eye medication from home with him.

When I saw George the next day at three o'clock in the afternoon, no eye medication had come, even though the nurse had ordered both of them. Immediately, I gave him the ones I brought from home, but I was exasperated. Apparently these meds were once again on special order. Weren't there ever any other people with glaucoma in the hospital?

Two more mistakes also come to mind that happened when George was in the hospital for a fractured hip. My cousin Leah alerted me that he was being given several blood tests. I questioned the nurse about it, and we discovered that the person who took his blood thought he was the patient who had previously been in the now empty bed next to him.

The blood test mistake was nothing compared to the second mistake that could have cost George his life. The surgeon and the anesthesiologist both failed to note important information on his entrance file. After George had fasted for many hours, the anesthesiologist came in his hospital room to talk with him before surgery. I thank God that I was there because I mentioned that George had a heart attack a few years ago and was now on blood thinner. The anesthesiologist seemed surprised and announced that this changed everything. He would need to get a release from the heart specialist for the surgery and also check the level of blood thinner in George's blood. This was not an easy thing for my stepfather since the next day he had to fast again for several more hours before the rescheduled surgery.

I was so upset about this that I took my compliant to the patient advocate that lead to a further interview with her boss. I was told the doctors should look at the patients' file, and yes, it was disturbing that he got the wrong blood tests.

A few weeks after George came home, a head nurse from the floor he had been on telephoned me. A positive change was made due to my complaint. She explained that a new procedure that included a double check had been instituted, so mistakes regarding blood tests would never happen again. Unfortunately, no mention was made about the oversight of George's surgeon and anesthesiologist that was the more serious of the two problems.

George was not the only one who suffered under poor hospital care. My mother came home from the hospital once with a horrible diaper rash. Another time she came home with a bedsore and a staph infection on the heel of her foot. It took about seven months of visiting the wound care center to heal it, and she had permanent tissue loss.

After all these problems, I made sure my parents didn't go to the hospital unless it was completely necessary and the last resort. When they absolutely had to be in the hospital, I was always checking to make sure nothing went wrong. I also continued to pray, asking my Heavenly Father to watch over my parents and give me wisdom. He went before us and came behind us. His protection was always with us even when we were unaware that we needed it.

YOUR JOURNAL

In what ways will you be an alert advocate if your loved one must go to the hospital?

TIP FOR CAREGIVER

I stored my parents' clothes and handkerchiefs that they used most often in the upper bureau drawers. Washcloths and kitchen towels that were needed constantly, I put on the most accessible shelves in the linen closet. Our caregiver and I placed my parents' pills in plastic weekly organizers that we kept on two different kitchen counters in plain view. Basically anything we used often was kept nearby and handy.

It Starts Again

It starts again.
He's back in that place.
How many times now?
I've lost count.

Again, I'll enter the cave
with armor and sword,
ready to defend him
against the dark warlocks
with white coats and wrong potions.

Outside vivid daffodils
and budding lilacs
must get along
without my applause
while the white wizard regulates
the thinness of his blood
and finally lets him go free.

Luke 8:11

"This is what the parable means: the seed is the word of God."

Luke 8:15

"The seeds that fell in good soil stand for those who hear the message and retain it in a good and obedient heart, and they persist until they bear fruit."

Praise for Christians Writers

There are many positive, encouraging, and uplifting Christian books based on the Word of God. While I was a caregiver to my parents, I was thankful for great books written by Joyce Meyer, Joel Osteen, Norman Vincent Peale, Rick Warren, Emilie Barnes, and Charles H. Spurgeon. The list of powerful Christian writers seems endless. These authors helped me apply the Bible to my own life and still do.

With prayer and these wonderful books, along with sermons that I heard on radio and television, I was able to find my way out of self-pity and sadness. Many times I had questions about something that was bothering me. Viola! There it was in something I read or heard in a sermon. God chose many ways to speak to me and teach me what I needed to know along the way.

*

Too often I complained about some of my duties such as changing Mom's diaper or balancing my parents' checkbook. These complaints reflected my true thoughts and feelings, but it also showed that I was dwelling too hard on the negative part of my job as caregiver. It was a problem for Bill too because he had to listen to me. This was not healthy situation for our marriage.

God must have wanted me to know there was a better way to deal with annoying tasks. Through two separate readings in Christian books and one Joyce Meyer radio program, all within a matter of a few days, God taught me that mature Christians should not whine and complain. *I understand,* I told God.

It was obvious to me that it wasn't going to be easy to give-up complaining since it was so ingrained in my thought pattern, but at least I would try to stop. I had to remind myself that my goal was to be a mature Christian. I had to pray for God's help in breaking this old bad habit. God would do His part, but I had do mine.

*

It amazed me how often the subject of my inspirational reading for the day was exactly what I needed at that moment. I shouldn't have been so surprised by this since God can do anything. If I was willing to listen and be open to His leading, God taught me what I needed to learn, and He still does.

Perhaps I was given the hard job of caregiver to my parents in order for my soul to grow closer to God. To make it through a hard day, I was encouraged to draw closer to my Heavenly Father for wisdom and guidance. I learned that the best way to get through any difficult trial in life is by praying often and waiting for God's answer to come. It does come; God is faithful.

YOUR JOURNAL

Have you heard or read something recently that was an answer to prayer? If not, is there something you want to ask God today?

TIP FOR CAREGIVER

Along the long windowsill in my parents' room, I placed a bunch of small potted African violets and inpatients. These plants flowered all winter. It was so cheerful to lift the shades in the morning and see flowers blooming while outside the trees were bare or full of snow. George couldn't see, and I wasn't sure if Mom noticed, but they certainly helped to lift my spirits.

Celebrating

The birdhouse in our apple tree is full again.
The wren sits . . . expectant
while her mate warbles incessantly
from outer branches.

The triple-colored cat has a big belly.
She yawns,
already half asleep
in a box lined with fleece.

My mother's arthritic finger circles
a picture of a toddler in a magazine.
Her lift-chair longs for a bath
while the television grows weary.

Stepfather's dialysis works another
miracle . . . secretly, quietly.
He comes home depleted,
dry as antique furniture.

My voice reaches Heaven.
God blows me a thought
for enthusiasm.
Joy comes by for a visit.

Again, I'm a new bell
clanging, clanging,
celebrating.
All is as it should be
in this life given to me.

Psalm 116:1-2

"I love the Lord, because he hears me;
   he listens to my prayers.
He listens to me
   every time I call to him."

Fun

During the years I was a caregiver, I looked forward to the times our assistant stayed with my parents for a few days, so Bill and I could take a five-hour car trip to visit our daughter Kelly, her husband Kurt and our grandson John. When I woke up in their guest room on an air mattress beside Bill, I was happy. I knew there was fun ahead, spending time with our family who we didn't get to see as often as we would have liked. It also meant Bill and I would have a chance to recharge and refresh ourselves before we returned home where commitment and responsibility waited for us.

During one visit, John and I worked hard on an art project. We both used colorful markers on black velvet pictures that I purchased at the craft store. He made one of space ships, space stations, and stars and another of a dragon fighter and a fiery dragon. Mine was a flowered heart shaped wreath with the word *love* across the front. When his pictures were finished, John helped me with mine. It made me feel good to find something that we both enjoyed and could do together.

I was able to get John two 12 x 20 frames at a reasonable price, so we could hang both his pictures on his playroom wall. My picture came home with me where it will always be a reminder of special time spent with my grandson.

*

Usually we headed back home on Sunday. This was always a difficult day for me. I often felt afraid and upset because back home there were seemingly a million things I had to do and worry about. There was the housework on our side and their side. There was the cooking for all of us. There was medication to keep track of and order. There were the trips to the doctor, and way too many trips to the emergency room. Also as soon as we returned, our assistant usually took a couple days off which meant I had full charge of my parents.

Just the thought of all this ahead made me want to give up being a caregiver, yet at the same time, I wanted to be in charge of making sure they were peaceful and as well as possible in their remaining years. These two opposing thoughts were always with me.

If I wanted to feel better, I discovered I needed to pray, asking God to give me enthusiasm for the work ahead. Also I would quote from the Bible: *This is the day the Lord has made; let us rejoice and be glad in it.* Saying this verse made me feel a bit happier and lighter inside

God knew it was extra hard for me to return home now that my parents were so helpless. Nevertheless again I would trust Him. Surely, He would guide me into an attitude of acceptance, but I had to do my part and not dwell on the negative.

YOUR JOURNAL

What fun things have you done lately or plan to do for yourself soon?

TIP FOR CAREGIVER

As my mother got weaker, her whole face seemed to disappear into the pillow when she was lying on her side. We worried that she might suffocate. In order to solve this problem, we used a firmer pillow that supported her cheek, so her nose and mouth cleared the pillow.

I Never Knew Till Now

Early, sometimes 5:30 AM, the baby monitor moans.
The warm bed holds me until I'm brave enough
to propel myself out into the cold.

Wrapping myself in fleece, I slide into slippers,
heading for the doors, connecting ours to theirs.

My child with big brown eyes and graying hair is awake.
Good-morning, I say. Sometimes there is a smile.
I hug her tight, but she weeps then laughs,
overcome by emotion.

Sitting bedside, I give her my hand.
She lifts it to her lips for a kiss. *See, I am a good mother.*

I love you, Mom, I say.
She understands enough to mumble the same.
I never knew till now the weight of my words.

John 15:12

"My commandment is this: love one another, just as I love you."

Rising Above

Suddenly George's congestive heart failure became serious, and we had to call 911. Following doctor's orders, we gave him more of the medication that clears fluid out of his lungs. This meant he was breathing easier even before the paramedics arrived.

He was in the hospital for three days before he came home in relatively good shape. Admittedly there was no way to know how long it would be before he would have another episode. The heart specialist warned me that eventually kidney dialysis and water pills would no longer work to keep his lung clear of fluid.

Now that George was back home, Bill, Jean, and I were on edge knowing he might need another trip to the hospital soon, but there was also something else that kept us alert. He began to do weird things with his walker. He often got up before it was in front of him, and he'd have to stretch his arm to reach it. Since his legs were weak, he could easily topple right over. At one point, he was confused and walked with it to the top of the stairs and just stood there. I don't want to think about what could have happened.

Another phenomenon was taking place that I knew happens to many elderly people when they become weak and tired. George needed to be encouraged to wash strategic areas of his body every day. If it were up to him, he would take a shower once a week and smell awful the rest of the time. It was only after I was probably too blunt about his lack of personal hygiene that he became more cooperative about keeping himself clean.

We also had to encourage him to eat, and to stay out of bed and awake as much as possible. Left to himself, he would not have gotten enough calories for good health. Also, he would have slept all day and been up all night, something he absolutely hated.

This last time that George was at the hospital, I believe God gave me this thought. *George won't live much longer. It is good to spend more time with him. My time is my final gift to him.*

Sometimes I did have a few saintly thoughts, but truthfully I still longed for more personal time and freedom from being a caregiver. Only with God's help and with the two people He provided to assist me, I would stay the course in this labor of love. I would spend more time with George, trying to keep him happy in his final months on earth.

I had learned that commitment doesn't always feel good, even though it might be the right thing to do. No matter how much I would have rather been somewhere else and doing something else, I still rose above these human desires and continued to care for my parents at home.

YOUR JOURNAL

If you were not a caregiver, what would you be doing instead? How do you feel about that?

TIP FOR CAREGIVER

With the high cost of oil, we kept the thermostat set between 67 to 70 degrees which was a little on the chilly side for my parents. They preferred 75 degrees all the time. Our assistant or I helped them dress in warm fleece, thermals, or a couple of layers of clothing if needed. During winter nights, they wore socks and soft fleece hats. On bitter cold days, they kept their hats on round-the-clock and felt warm and cozy under one of my mother's many knitted and crocheted lap blankets.

Service

There is something disconcerting about a lift-chair
left upright.
It's like the door needing a shove,
crumpled sheets needing a tug,
shoelaces needing a tie,
pots needing a scrub.

The upright chair waits for my mother's return,
while I wait for freedom—
even though it comes with a catch.
No analgesic will numb the wound
except the cliché of time.

I stand there looking at the lift-chair,
its arms out, suspended . . . waiting.
How long? I wonder.
But the chair cannot choose its beloved
or try on the slippers of a saint.

Proverbs 18:13

"Listen before you answer. If you don't, you are being stupid and insulting."

A Lesson

The last time George was in the hospital, I was reminded of something that I thought I learned a long time ago. Nurses and techs at the hospital only react quickly to someone bleeding or not being able to breathe. The majority of the time they give patients the right medication at the appropriate time, but basically, everything else comes slowly. Sometimes what I wanted done for George or Mom, I had to do myself. Nurses and aides are extremely busy, so this is the way it is.

On Monday evening, I had left a request with George's nurse that he needed help washing up, but at lunchtime the next day, I noticed that his clean underwear was still in there. To me this meant he had not washed. I was angry. This poor man at ninety-five had fragile skin that became irritated if he wasn't clean, not to mention the awful smell.

I asked George if he was washed, and he said yes. Well then, now I really was angry and basically hit the ceiling, at least my voice did. I ranted and raved like a lunatic, saying, *They washed him and didn't change his underwear?* The nurse was with the patient in the next bed over. Behind the closed curtain she answered me by saying, *I can hear you.* Of course, she did. Everyone in the hospital heard me. Then the tech came. She tried to tell me something, but I wouldn't let her speak. I was all rived-up and totally out of control.

Finally, finally, I listened. The tech explained that she told George she would return to wash his bottom. He hadn't told me that part. Then I turned around and yelled at him. I had allowed my frustration of not being able to control what was happening in the hospital get the best of me.

After George finished eating, I told him I'd be back around 4 PM. As I walked to the car, I berated myself for being so out of control. I had overreacted. I was a fool to make a mountain out of a molehill. I had been a horrible Christian example.

Again I am reminded that I am a branch and must stay firmly attached to vine, my Lord and Savior Jesus. I cannot bear fruit on my own. I must draw nutrients from the vine in order to produce good fruit. This means that next time I go to the hospital I need to pray and ask for patience ahead of time.

I also must remind myself that the nurses and techs are extremely busy, most of the time doing the best they can for many people. Only priority concerns can get addressed immediately.

YOUR JOURNAL

Do you remember a time when you became angry before listening to the whole story? If not, what is your secret?

TIP FOR CAREGIVER

My parents' doctor told me that elderly people do not feel the heat in the summer. That is why so often we hear in the news about some elderly person dying from heatstroke. The doctor said in order to prevent heat related problems, we should use an air conditioner and offer my parents sweaters to keep warm.

Since George had kidney and congestive heart failure, he was prone to breathing problems, especially when it was hot and humid. The higher electric bill could not be a factor in our decision whether to run the AC. It helped George breathe easier, so it was a necessity rather than a luxury.

Please Listen

When the alarm misses it's calling,
    the coffee pot has a nervous breakdown,
        the to-do-list is three pages long,
            the computer doesn't know you,
                the refrigerator hums its swan song,
                    the microwave turns a cold shoulder,
                      the car says *service engine soon*,
                          the dog piddles on the floor,
                          the TV plays dead,
                              and everyone drops the
                              ball

please listen to Jesus
because His words can
soothe your soul and
bring peace
in an instant.

Ephesians 6:13-18a

"So put on God's armor now! Then when the evil day comes, you will be able to resist the enemy's attacks; and after fighting to the end, you will still hold your ground.

So stand ready, with truth as a belt tight around your waist, with righteousness as your breastplate, and as your shoes the readiness to announce the Good News of peace. At all times carry faith as a shield; for with it you will be able to put out all the burning arrows shot by the Evil One. And accept salvation as a helmet, and the word of God as the sword which the Spirit gives you. Do all this in prayer, asking for God's help."

Christians Get Upset Too

Stephen Ministries is an organization of church members especially trained to support people who are going through a crisis in their lives. Our son Keith who teaches this program explained to me that some Christians may suffer more during hard times than nonbelievers because they might worry that something must be wrong with their relationship with God if they are unhappy. Of course, this may not be true at all. I already understood this concept, but it made me feel better to hear it again.

Sometimes it was hard to imagine that God wanted me to continue caring for my parents at home since way too often I felt trapped and sad. While at the same time, I also felt led by God to continue this commitment. I understood that even though this work made me unhappy from time to time, it did not necessarily mean I was on the wrong path. It only meant that I was doing an extremely difficult job that would be a challenge for anyone.

When I was tired of feeling sorry for myself, I would say to myself, *Yes, this is hard, and I wish I didn't have to do it, but I still can see this commitment through to the end. God will give me the strength and enthusiasm that I need each day. He will not give me what I need a week from now or even a day from now, only what I need today. That is enough.*

YOUR JOURNAL

When you need to hear positive thoughts, what do you tell yourself?

TIP FOR CAREGIVER

Often when I made my parents' beds, I would place cheery throw pillows on them. Till this day, I still have these pillows and continue to use them. One has a picture of a patio with flowers and a comfy rocking chair with the words, *Welcome each new day*. Another has a picture of garden where two ladies are sitting side by side in a chair with the words: *Sisters are blossoms in the garden of life*. These pillows decorated the room of a blind man and a mother with dementia, but at least it made me happy that my parents' room looked comfortable and inviting.

Heartsick

He leads the way to the place
where we put last year's leaves.
There a fawn with spots is sleeping
while its mother grazes nearby
with no guarantee of safety since

nature can be cruel.
One spring a crow in search of meat
overturned a robin's nest in our cherry tree.
Bill repositioned a chick on the branch,
but there was only one to save.

As we walk back to our front door,
I am heartsick and wonder why
caring for my elderly parents makes me sad.
The wind gives me a little nudge as if to say,
Remember, this isn't heaven yet.

Matthew 26:39

"He [Jesus] went a little farther on, threw himself face downward on the ground, and prayed, 'My Father, if it is possible, take this cup of suffering from me! Yet not what I want, but what you want.'"

A Weak Attempt

One morning, I read some pages of Rick Warren's book, *The Purpose Driven Life*. I was reminded that I needed to surrender to God's will; on this day, however, like so many others, my spirit felt weak. I could not whole-heartedly embrace the sacrifice of caring for my parents, and I prayed that this commitment would end. If it was God's will that I continue this work, I wanted to do it, but then again, I didn't want to do it. I was full of contradictions, but each day I continued to watch over my parents anyway, making sure they were safe and secure.

Maybe this ambivalence was just part of being human. After all, Rick Warren did remind me that Jesus prayed for His sacrifice to be taken from Him, and at the same time, He also prayed for God's will to be done. I couldn't pray with the same purity and sincerity as Jesus, but I would offer my weak attempt anyway.

YOUR JOURNAL

Is there anything you wish you didn't have to do, but you do it anyway?

TIP FOR CAREGIVER

As my mother's mobility decreased and her circulation worsened, sores became a constant threat. They first began when she developed an antibiotic resistant infection in her right heel during a hospital stay. Then due to poor circulation, she later developed other more serious wounds. I came to understand that when sores are hard to heal, only the experts of at a wound care center know how to treat them.

Only Human

We hug them in the morning,
longing for their bedtime.
We wash their clothes,
wearing ours wrinkled.
We drive them everywhere,
trapping ourselves.
We cook them mashed potatoes,
stuffing our faces with chips.
We give them a bath,
wishing for time alone.
We tell them funny stories,
feeling sorry for ourselves.
We kiss them goodnight,
wanting our place in the sun.
We are only human,
trying to love.

Romans 8:28

"We know that in all things God works for good with those who love him, those whom he has called according to his purpose."

Critical Importance

I had a horrible sinking feeling in the pit of my stomach, thinking what could have happened. Earlier that day, I had brought my mother outside in her wheelchair on the deck of our house, and I left her in the sun, thinking I'll be back in ten minutes to move her into the shade. She ended up being in full sun for thirty minutes because I got distracted. A good thing she had a deep olive complexion because otherwise she would have gotten badly burned. Her skin did get red and hot, but after I put her in the shade and gave her a cool drink she was fine.

Our assistant and I continued to learn many important lessons while we took care of my elderly parents. On this day, I had learned something of critical importance. My mother could not be left in the sun while I went back inside the house. It was just too dangerous.

YOUR JOURNAL

What have you learned recently?

TIP FOR CAREGIVER

Before my parents developed serious medical problems, Bill and I would take them for little outings. When George felt up to it, he and I would go to church together. My mother enjoyed car rides; she loved to watch the world go by. All four of us went to restaurants, just to get out and to give me a break from cooking. Once we shared four different meals, buffet style. On the way home from a doctor's appointment, we all enjoyed hamburgers at a fast food restaurant or an ice cream cones at a neighborhood convenience store. We also visited family, people that my mother and George enjoyed seeing. These many outings gave all of us a change in scenery and a lift to our spirits.

Out of Body

Sometimes on a busy day,
part of me goes away,
speeding off in a car,
traveling somewhere much too far.
What's left goes through all the motions,
working with those empty notions,
never really quite all there
until reality gives a scare.

I cook and then burn the pot.
My Mom in the hot sun, I forgot.
On dialysis day it's a crime;
I don't get Stepfather out on time.
I am glad no one's been hurt.
God's protection did not desert.

Shaking my head, I realize,
it's a matter of focus, no surprise.
As nurse, wife, and maid,
my wayward half I must persuade
to stop gallivanting all around
and come straight back into town.

I catch a taxi, the first I see,
hop a train to Station Z,
and ride a bike to the beach.
Out of breath I finally reach
the dreamer resting in the sun.
Then I yell, *Vacation's done!*
Reunited we travel home
with an order not to roam.

Now I must concentrate,
most mistakes irradiate.
Today after the work is done,
that is when I'll have some fun.

Psalm 112:6

"A good person will never fail;
he will always be remembered."

I Can't Do It Alone

Bill will be away. Our assistant will be here to help with my parents. Now I won't have to cook big meals since my parents are satisfied with something simple. Also, I won't be spending time with Bill in the evening, watching television. I'll have some free time to do my writing and my crafting. Wrong!

Without Bill to drive George to dialysis, I discovered I had much less time to myself. It took up a large chunk of my time, bringing George to dialysis, waiting for him to get through, and then bringing him back home.

While Bill was away, I was reminded never to take my dear husband for granted because he was as important as my right hand. Without his help and support I would be too busy and too tired to go on caring for my parents at home. I would try to remember to thank him often.

YOUR JOURNAL

Who is the person in your life who makes your job possible?

TIP FOR CAREGIVER

When my mother had the wound on the heel of her foot, the wound care center encouraged us to use heel protectors. These foam boots suspended both kneels over air, protecting the area against pressure that in turn increased blood circulation. Without adequate blood circulation the wound would not heal or could become worse. Of course, there were places that defied being suspended in air, such as the bottom of her spine and buttock, but for those areas, we were instructed to rotate her position often.

Responsibility

Today, I don't want to be good.
I'm just too tired.
I want to stay under the covers
and hide myself from Responsibility.
But Responsibility tickles my neck
with a soft finger,
kisses me on the forehead
with warm lips,
and with a quiet voice
tells me I am needed.
Oka-a-a-y, I say,
dragging myself out of bed.

I Corinthians 13:1-7

"I may be able to speak the languages of human beings and even of angels, but if I have no love, my speech is no more than a noisy gong or a clanging bell. I may have the gift of inspired preaching; I may have all knowledge and understand all secrets; I may have all the faith needed to move mountains—but if I have no love, I am nothing. I may give away everything I have, and even give up my body to be burned—but if I have no love, this does me no good.

Love is patient and kind; it is not jealous or conceited or proud; love is not ill-mannered or selfish or irritable; love does not keep a record of wrongs; love is not happy with evil, but is happy with the truth. Love never gives up; and its faith, hope, and patience never fail."

The Most Loving Way

Bill and I traveled home from Maine after another visit with our daughter and her family. On our first full day back, our assistant was supposed to have off, but she kindly offered to come in between 3 PM and 6 PM. While I cooked, she looked after my parents. Later she would feed my mother her supper and get her ready for bed. I always appreciated our assistant being here, especially after our short vacations when it took me a day or two to adjust back into the responsibility and work of being a caregiver.

On the second day back from our trip, I still was off kilter. While I was caring for my mother, I became impatient with George. The tone of my voice must have given away my negative feelings. George said he wanted to go back to bed because he didn't want to be in the way and give me more work. Of course, right away I understood my mistake. I hugged him, saying that he wasn't in the way. I explained that I had been busy with my mother and not able to assist him immediately. He seemed to feel better, and he didn't go to bed.

This little episode, which sadly happened on Father's Day, made me realize I had to be more patient. Occasionally, I actually caught myself trying to make George feel bad. This was totally unacceptable because I couldn't do the best for him or my mother unless I did it lovingly. No matter how I felt, I had to talk with them with kindness.

*

Sometimes I found myself thinking that it would be best to put my parents in a nursing home. Then I would quit thinking these thoughts, since I believed that God wanted me to keep my parents at home with Bill and me. It was the best way I could keep them as happy as possible and safe in their remaining years.

By no means do I criticize others who must turn to nursing homes for their parents. Some people do not have the monetary resources for an assistant, the extra space in their house, and a supportive spouse, relative or friend that I had. It is my opinion that success as a home caregiver comes more easily if all three of these ingredients are present. If anything had changed my situation, I too would have needed to place my parents in a nursing home.

YOUR JOURNAL

Are you at peace with being an at-home caregiver? If not, why?

TIP FOR CAREGIVER

When the wound care center made us realize that another key step in avoiding bedsores was the use of a high quality moisturizer, I compared products. I was able to find a less expensive generic moisturizer with the same ingredients as the well-known, more expensive brand.

Used to Be

It used to be safe here, but
last night a bear yanked down
our bird feeder, straightening
the heavy metal hook.
Now shadows in the yard
make me nervous.

There used to be room for store plants.
Now the ferns grow close to our house.
They unfurl as if they belong here;
maybe they do.

My parents used to be my support system.
Now I help him get dressed, and
she is a toddler, not yet toilet trained.

I used to think love was kind words.
How naive I was back then
in my days of seesaws and swings.

Now I choose commitment,
sliding forward with no way back, but
why do I kick and scream all the way down,
Please, God, don't let the sacrifice be me.

Philippians 2:13

" . . . God is always at work in you to make you willing and able to obey his own purpose."

An Unpleasant Job

George was short of breath every time he walked just a few short steps. He had been on oxygen at night, but now he also had to use portable oxygen during the day. It was a huge effort for him to take a shower or shave. He already had a few episodes of congestive heart failure, landing him in the hospital. His heart doctor warned me that eventually dialysis and water pills would not keep enough fluid out of his lungs.

Even though George had become extremely weak, there was one thing I never wanted to do for him. *I will never wipe my stepfather's bottom*, I had said many times to Bill and our assistant. It was bad enough I had to do it for my mother, but for my stepfather I would draw the line.

God had something else in mind. The day came when George couldn't wipe his own bottom after using the toilet. I found myself doing what I said I would never do. It was either do it or put him in a nursing home immediately which I didn't want to do. At first this chore was a bit embarrassing, probably more so for George than me, but somehow we are both got beyond that.

God wanted me to grow and mature in ways I could never have imagined. Again I was reminded that sometimes love is not just flowery, good feelings. In some cases, when we are called by God to help one of his children, the job is hard and unpleasant.

This noble thought did not magically make me happy about caring for George. It was a job that seemed to be getting harder and harder by the minute. It was a challenge to say the least, especially on dialysis days and when our assistant had off from work.

I had to get George out of bed, help him dress, give him breakfast, set him up with his portable oxygen, and with Bill's help get him down the chairlift on the stairs and into the car.

On these same mornings, with Bill's assistance, I got my mother out of bed into her wheelchair and put her on the toilet. I'd clean her up and dress her, and then Bill would put her back into the wheelchair and transfer her into the chair in the living room. Without Bill's help, there was no way I could have done all this before he and George left for dialysis. My back just would not have tolerated the heavy lifting, and my emotions would not have tolerated the stress.

YOUR JOURNAL

Is there a job you hope you will never have to do as a caregiver?

TIP FOR CAREGIVER

My mother often rubbed her eyes which were prone to infection. I tried to keep her hands extra clean throughout the day by using antibacterial hand wipes and rinsing with wet paper towels. This was a convenient alternative to soap and water at the sink.

Looking Back

How do those tiny wrens work all day,
finding food for their young?
How do they sing so richly?
How do they survive thunderstorms that
shake the trees?

How did I watch my parents become
old and frail?
How did I ride the ambulance with them
so many times I lost count?

1 Peter 5:6-7

"Humble yourselves, then, under God's mighty hand, so that he will lift you up in his own good time. Leave all your worries with him, because he cares for you."

A Decision to Stop Fighting

Bill and I were not home when George had trouble breathing again and our assistant had to call 911. After we got home, our assistant explained that when help arrived, George refused to go to the hospital, saying he wanted to die at home. He also told her that he did not want to go to dialysis anymore.

When I went into the bedroom to see him, he was breathing easier. He made it clear to me that he would not go to dialysis anymore. This meant that he would die within a few days. Immediately, I called hospice, thinking I would need their support right away. A very kind nurse said that the offices were closed, but tomorrow I could sign him in.

After this telephone call, George had trouble breathing again. He told me that he thought he should go to the hospital, but he wasn't sure what to do. He wanted me to decide.

I explained hospice could not help us immediately, and I thought he should go to the hospital where he could get medication that would keep him comfortable. My words made sense to him, and we called for an ambulance. At the hospital, he was hooked up to oxygen which helped him to breathe easier.

I wondered if he would change his mind about dialysis the next day. His doctor would order this procedure for him at the hospital if this is what George wanted.

*

When George decided not to go to dialysis, my internal state could have been summed up in one word, *GUILT!* I had spoken to my stepfather at least three times about how he had a choice; he didn't have to keep going to dialysis. The subject came up once when he mentioned he wanted to die. Another time it was when he refused food, and my patience was wearing thin. A part of me was sure he would never stop going, but I was wrong. Now he was taking my advice. It sent guilt waves like knives right through me.

Was it something I said? I asked him.

It's my decision, he said.

I'll take care of you forever, I told him.

Even though he still insisted this was what he wanted, my feeling of guilt would not go away, because I knew in my heart I was tired of taking care of him and a part of me wanted him to die. My motive for discussing his options had not been pure.

George had become helpless, needing assistance on and off the toilet, washing, and dressing. Our assistant or I had to monitor his fluid intake, closely. This was extremely stressful for him as well as for us since he always wanted more fluid than was recommended by his doctor. I worried constantly about what I could give him to eat that was low in sodium yet palatable. Most of the time, he was not hungry and I worried about that too. It was hard trying to keep him awake during the day in the hope he would have a restful night. I tried to be kind, but I must admit I hated it when he rang his little bell in the middle of the night. I would have to force myself out of my bed to give him a sleeping pill or help him out of his bed so he could go to the bathroom.

All this worry and work was physically tiring and emotionally draining. This was my only excuse for wishing that I didn't want to take care of George any more. I intensely regretted telling him that he could stop dialysis. What kind of monster had I become? I wondered if I should have put my parents in a nursing home before it had come to this.

I reminded myself that I told George that I would take care of him forever. I also knew that his mind was sound. It was his choice to stop living, yet it took a long time before I could forgive myself.

YOUR JOURNAL

Have you ever said anything to your loved one that you are sorry about or wish you could have said more kindly?

TIP FOR CAREGIVER

Looking back, I should have encouraged my parents to meet with a financial planner while my mother still had a clear mind. Without this type of planning, their life savings would have vanished if they needed to go into a nursing home. As it turned out, we needed to spend a hefty portion of their savings for an assistant anyway, but at least they got the best possible care.

Four Years of Dialysis

The machine, the cleaning machine,
washed his blood three times a week.
The machine, the hurting machine,
punctured his artery with a thick needle.
The machine, the imperfect machine,
no longer cleared his lungs of fluid.
The machine, the manmade machine,
will keep someone else alive
now that he's gone.

John 3:16-17

"For God loved the world so much that he gave his only Son, so that everyone who believes in him may not die but have eternal life. For God did not send his Son into the world to be its judge, but to be its savior."

Last Days

Before George went into the hospital, he insisted that it was his decision to stop kidney dialysis. From his hospital bed, he told me that he was thankful for all Bill and I had done for him and that he would miss me. I told him I would miss him too, but I understood why he made this decision.

Every morning his doctor asked George if he wanted to change his mind and have a dialysis treatment. Every morning he said, no.

George had been in the hospital three and a half days. He became weaker, but continued to have a clear mind. He spoke at length to the pastor of his church. He even ate a few handfuls of peanuts that I brought from home.

His kidney doctor told the nurse that he thought George would die this day. I prayed for God's guidance whether to stay through the night.

It was early evening when his breathing became strained. I asked the nurse if he could have some morphine; this would ease the strain of trying to breathe. She notified the doctor, and within minutes, he was on a morphine drip. I knew the end was near. At some point, he called out my name. He wanted to know if I was still there. I responded that I was. Clearly, he wanted me there.

Even though he was on the morphine drip, he still couldn't sleep, so he asked for his usual sleeping pill. The nurse explained to me that it would be hard for him to swallow now that he was on the morphine, but I told her he was insisting on a pill to help him sleep. With some difficulty he did get the pill down. He closed his eyes and eventually became unresponsive when the nurse called out his name. Later when he appeared to be struggling for air again, I asked the nurse to increase his morphine, and she complied. George seemed peaceful again.

In the wee hours of Monday morning, while I sat in a chair on the other side of the room, writing some notes, he quietly passed away. *God bless his soul.* It had been sad to watch him die, but this was what he wanted. At ninety-five, he was tired, and he had no fight left in him.

George believed he would go to a better place; Paradise he called it. I had faith that he was already there, happy and completely well.

I called Bill to tell him that George had passed, and he called Pastor Gloria. She had been coming to the hospital twice a day to talk with George, and now she came to pray with me over his body. She asked if I wanted her to stay with him until the funeral home picked him up, but I said no.

He's not here. He's in heaven now, I told her.

She seemed pleased with my response.

My prayers had been answered. George died peacefully. I am glad I stayed with him all night, making sure he was comfortable.

*

Since I didn't hear from George's kidney doctor, I called him the next day to thank him. He had taken care of George and had worked with our assistant and me for almost three years. He had made sure George's passing was peaceful by ordering the morphine. It made me feel good to thank him, and he seemed to appreciate my call.

YOUR JOURNAL

Have you ever thought of thanking a doctor, nurse, or health care provider for their good care of your loved one? What would you say?

TIP FOR CAREGIVER

The wound care center suggested we buy special bandages that aid in the healing of sores. Sometimes the bandages needed to be changed every few days and sometimes more often, depending on the location of the wound. These hi-tech bandages and material for packing the wounds are extremely costly. My husband discovered that ordering them from an Internet company is less expensive than the local pharmacies.

Undecided

I walk in our yard
where the grass grows and
winter is undecided.
Warm temperatures makes
the forsythia bush think
it might be time to bloom.
Daffodils wave their
green question marks
in the air.

If anyone understands winter's
dilemma, it is me.
Stepfather passed away, and
I still don't know if I love him.
Perhaps keeping him alive
with tender-loving-care
and oxygen was only duty.

Yet I am certain,
if he appeared in his chair
munching peanuts,
I'd give him a quick kiss
on his greasy forehead
before he left me again.

Philippians 3:12-14

"I do not claim that I have already succeeded or have already become perfect. I keep striving to win the prize for which Christ Jesus has already won me to himself. Of course, my friends, I really do not think that I have already won it; the one thing I do, however, is to forget what is behind me and do my best to reach what is ahead. So I run straight toward the goal in order to win the prize, which is God's call through Christ Jesus to the life above."

God Before Me and Behind Me

    Lots of pressure was off Bill and me. We no longer worried that at a moment's notice we would find ourselves on the way to the hospital because George couldn't breathe again. Now we had more time because we did not have to transport him back and forth to dialysis. It was good not to have so much work to do, but the house seemed empty without George. He was always a good listener if I needed someone to talk to, and he had a good sense of humor. His decision for himself had been right though. Just breathing had become difficult for him, and he was always weak and tired. Now he didn't have to suffer any more.

*

    I shouldn't have been so amazed that my Father in Heaven went before me and came behind me during this hard time. After all, His wisdom, power, and love are greater than I can ever comprehend. I was still awed that He had taught me something just before I needed it.

    I had read Joyce Meyer's book, *In Pursuit of Peace, 21 Ways to Conquer Anxiety, Fear, and Discontentment*. The ninth chapter of this book is titled "Accept Yourself." God knew that shortly I would need these comforting words. Meyer writes, "We struggle and strive for perfection, but somehow it eludes us. Our pursuit is in vain." She also writes, "We are new spiritual clay. We are being shaped into perfection, but not there yet." She explains that we can have peace anyway because God made us perfect and righteous in Christ. This chapter reminded me that God forgave me for my wrong motives when I suggested to George that he stop going to dialysis.

Now it was my turn to forgive myself. I knew if I didn't forgive myself and continued to torture myself then the devil would win. He wanted me to become mentally ill and unable to let the Holy Spirit work through me. No, I would not let this happen. God wanted me to forgive myself and move on to be a strong Christian in His service. He wanted me to smile and have joy in my heart because His Son died for my sins, and I am forgiven and loved.

YOUR JOURNAL

When you need forgiveness, what is your first step? After this first step are you able to forgive yourself?

TIP FOR CAREGIVER

The staff at the wound care center and a nutritionist, who came to speak with us at our home, helped our assistant and me understand the importance of a healthy diet in those people who have wounds. Certain vitamins and adequate protein are essential for the healing process. We were informed that there are special nutritional drinks made just for people with wounds.

These drinks with high protein, vitamins, and minerals soon became an important supplement to my mother's diet. Since George's appetite was not what it once was, we also gave him these special drinks. He called them milkshakes because it did taste that good. A few times I had one of these drinks when I was in a hurry and didn't want to buy a meal on the road.

Water

God's love is like water constantly dripping
against a hollow rock until it creates a pinhole of faith.
Each drop expands the opening until
a flood of water enters, washing all fear away.

Matthew 7:7-11

"Ask, and you will receive; seek, and you will find; knock, and the door will be opened to you. For everyone who asks will receive, and anyone who seeks will find, and the door will be opened to those who knock. Would any of you who are fathers give your son a stone when he asks for bread? Or would you give him a snake when he asks for fish? As bad as you are, you know how to give good things to your children. How much more, then, will your Father in heaven give good things to those who ask him!"

God' Guidance

Not again. I couldn't believe that so shortly after my stepfather's passing in September, we would be faced with another serious medical problem in December, yet here it was happening again.

It was only two months since George's death when my mother caught a virus that gave her cold symptoms and a fever. If she were a younger person, our assistant and I would have let the virus run its course and hope for the best, but instead we requested an antibiotic from her doctor. We hoped this would protect her from a secondary bacterial infection that might threaten her life.

Two weeks later, she appeared well, but she continued to have a wicked cough. We called her doctor asking for prescription cough medication, hoping this would be our answer. It turned out to be a big mistake.

The cough medication dried the mucus and allowed her to sleep, but it caused the return of her severe constipation problem. Since she had this difficulty on and off for years, we knew she was in trouble when her belly became huge. We stopped the cough medication with the result of the cough returning full force, but this was the least of her problems. Her skin color became pale, and we could tell she was uncomfortable. Our assistant and I took her to the ER and eventually she was admitted with possible pneumonia and stool impaction.

In one day, they were able to clear the impaction problem with liquid medication that is often used to prepare people for colonoscopies; however, the cough remained. Her doctor wasn't positive she had pneumonia, but treated her for it anyway. The first antibiotic caused a raised red area on her throat. I was the one who noticed it and brought to the nurse's attention. Apparently Mom was having an allergic reaction.

A good thing I was also there and alert to protest when they brought in another antibiotic. It was one that some time ago had given her an allergic reaction when she had been treated for an infection at home. I was upset because the warning that she was allergic to this antibiotic was on her wristband and in her hospital chart.

Finally an appropriate antibiotic was found, but it was not totally benign. The more medication she received intravenously, the groggier and weaker she became. It became more and more difficult for Bill, our assistant, or me to feed her because she was just too sleepy. It occurred to me that she might die.

The doctor ordered a swallowing test that I was not surprised showed trace amounts of barium had remained in her throat. This meant she could choke on her food and liquids. She could also develop aspiration pneumonia, caused by food entering her lungs. The doctor offered the option to have a g-tube placed in her stomach for feeding purposes.

I couldn't believe it. Just before my mother entered the hospital, she was eating and drinking just fine and now she needed a feeding tube? How could this be? I immediately said, *No*. This was quite unusual for me since I trust that most doctors know the right course of action when it comes to medical issues. However, now that my mother was elderly, my main concern for her was quality of life rather than quantity of days. I wanted her remaining time to be as peaceful and pleasant as possible. The feeding tube didn't seem to fit in this scenario.

I prayed about this decision and within a day or two, I felt a sense of peace about it. Bill and our assistant thought I made the right decision. We all were hoping that once Mom was off the antibiotic and back home, she would probably become stronger and perhaps overcome the swallowing difficultly.

*

Immediately after I made the decision for no G-tube, it was suggested to me by her doctor that I might want to put my mother under hospice care. This was a bit upsetting to me since a patient under this type of care is thought to have six months or less to live. Still I agreed to sign her in, thinking Bill, our assistant, and I needed all the help and guidance we could get.

Just before my mother was released from the hospital, a lady from hospice came to visit with us. I was pleased to hear a nurse would come to our home on a regular basis. Hopefully, the nurse would guide us how we could keep her as well and comfortable as possible. Also I would feel more secure, knowing I had someone to answer medical questions that might come up.

Little did I know that in the very near future I would be sorry that I registered Mom with hospice. In the end, the experience turned out to hurt her more than help her.

YOUR JOURNAL

What are your thoughts on quality of life versus quantity of life for those who are elderly or extremely ill?

TIP FOR CAREGIVER

My mother's wound care physician warned us that a bedsore can develop overnight, and it was essential to use an alternating air mattress on her bed. This type of mattress constantly changes pressure points on the body that allows for better blood circulation.

A few times we couldn't get a replacement right away for a deflated alternating air mattress. One of these delays caused my mother to develop another wound. Now I knew firsthand how urgent it was for her to have a good quality alternating air mattresses, and how important it was for me to check it often, making sure there were no leaks.

If She Could Talk To You

You say, *she might choke*
if allowed to chew.
She needs a feeding tube.
This is the safest move.

But just days ago,
she ate all man could grow.
She's always in that seat;
her one joy is to eat.
If she could talk to you,
she'd say, *I'll chance it to chew*
savory, homemade stew.

Proverbs 3:5-6

"Trust in the Lord with all your heart. Never rely on what you think you know. Remember the Lord in everything you do, and he will show you the right way."

Stronger

After ten days in the hospital, my mother was finally released but not before another mistake was almost made. Her doctor wrote a prescription for a continuation of an antibiotic by mouth at home. Only problem, it was the very same antibiotic that caused her to have red swelling on her neck. When the nurse called the doctor to alert him of the mistake, he decided not to give my mother another antibiotic at all. This did not make sense to me at all.

At home, it took another twenty-four hours before Mom was somewhat alert, and she began to get stronger. The cough persisted though, especially at night. She really couldn't get any good sleep and neither could we, listening to her.

Bill thought it would be a good idea, to bring her to an ear, nose, and throat doctor. I reluctantly agreed, thinking it would not help.

*

After we gave this new doctor my mother's recent medical history, and after he observed her drooling onto her coat bits of the breakfast she had just eaten, he had a diagnosis. She had poor swallowing along with acid reflux. He explained that swallowing problems, acid reflux, and impaction problems all come with end-stage dementia. He didn't think he could offer us much help, but he did give us a prescription for medication that would cut down acid production in her stomach. He suggested we give her smaller meals (more if necessary), make sure she did not lie down in bed after a meal for at least three hours, and he said a humidifier in her room was a good idea.

My mother was better the first night we followed the doctor's directions. We kept her in her chair after supper for three hours before putting her in bed. We also stopped giving her liquid stool softener as well because we read on the bottle that it could irritate the throat. We didn't over stuff her stomach with food, and we ran a humidifier in her room. That night was the first time she hardly coughed at all, and Bill and I also got a good night's sleep.

After just a little more than a week at home, my mother was back to herself, talking up a storm even though most of the time we didn't understand her. She was wide-awake during the day and smiled often, yet her much shorter bouts of coughing throughout the day and night reminded us she still had acid reflux.

My mother was back to eating everything; however, we did grind her meat and vegetables, and we also gave her thickened liquids to aide in the swallowing process. Perhaps she was at risk for choking or getting aspiration pneumonia, but I believed she would have agreed with my decision against the feeding tube.

YOUR JOURNAL

How will you go about making an important decision for your loved one if necessary?

TIP FOR CAREGIVER

Doctors often seem compelled to offer all medical options available. When I asked, however, what they would decide for their own frail and elderly parent, some indicated they would turn down the treatment they just offered. Most doctors choose quality of life over quantity and comfort over aggressive treatment. The key question to ask a doctor is *what would you do?*

Pluck

The dog can hardly walk, but still wags his tail.
The old tree stump grows new shoots.
Stepfather walks the day after hip surgery.

No more do I cling to expected ways.
A G-tube might keep Mother alive,
but she still eats hamburgers and apple pie.

Ecclesiastes 3:1-2a

"Everything that happens in this world happens at the time God chooses.

He sets the time for birth and the time for death . . ."

Not Again

Our happiness that my mother was improving soon turned back to discouragement. It was clear to us that her impaction problem never really left her. During the month since my mother had been home from the hospital, I had to give her double doses of strong laxatives about four times. Then I gave her medication that should have worked, but it did not. I wondered if she would ever have a BM again, and I feared that all these chemicals might eventually kill her.

Our assistant and I gave my mother a prescription laxative, fiber in her drinks, stool softener, and a high fiber diet each day. At least we did all that we could. I reminded myself it was ultimately in God's hands whether my mother lived or died, regardless of how I felt about it, regardless how much I oversaw her diet. Of course, in God's hands is always the best place to be.

*

I prayed that God would not allow my mother to suffer. Of course, I did not want to suffer either. Even though I was a good daughter who loved my mother, I have to admit it was hard for me to think of caring for her much longer. Too often I felt overwhelmed by responsibility and worry. Still I continued to find some peace by believing that God was in charge, and He alone decides matters of life and death.

YOUR JOURNAL

Would you be more peaceful if you put your loved one in God's hands and left him or her there?

TIP FOR CAREGIVER

I always say the bathroom and the kitchen are the two places that need to be neat and clean. I am in a better frame of mind, if these rooms sparkle and I can find things, not to mention a much smaller germ population.

Our assistant, Bill, and I took turns cleaning and straightening my parents' kitchen after meals and running the dishwasher at least once a day. If we put the clean dishes back in the cabinets early in the morning, then the dishwasher was free for the dirty ones, preventing a pile-up in the sink.

The Winter Blessing

For more than a month,
Mother seemed near death, but
for the time being, it appears she will live.
This morning my sore knee
threatens to keep me inside till spring.

I can't go to church, I moan.
Let's go, he says, nudging me out of bed.

We sneak in the back pew at the first hymn.
By the last stanza, the defrosting begins.
Next the pastor's words are the warm zephyr,
breathing life into my soul.

The sun leans in
against the windowpane,
listening to the sermon.
Its fingers pass
through the glass
to massage by my back.
Finally I remember
God's benevolence.

Proverbs 23:22

"Listen to your father; without him you would not exist. When your mother is old, show her your appreciation."

Hope and Worry

After taking my mother to the gastroenterologist, there was hope again. He put her on a new prescription laxative called Amitizia along with stool softeners. In fact, it worked so well, she was getting diarrhea. We had to cut back her daily dose to one every second day.

Then we realized we had cut back too much. Even though we quickly reverted back to the full dose, it happened again, no BM in three days. I prayed for guidance, and remembered the herbal laxative tea had helped another time. This time a strong cup of it did not produce results by her bedtime.

The next morning, I instructed our assistant to call the doctor early, but in the AM we were pleasantly surprised with a normal BM. It was truly a blessing, and I thanked God. I found it amazing how something as simple as this can make me so happy. Now I hoped my mother's care would finally go back to being somewhat manageable although there were other medical concerns.

Mom continued to have two wounds on her buttocks that required attention from the wound care center. These pressure sores, just like the others she had in the past, would be extremely hard to heal due to her poor circulation and inactivity.

Since she could not move on her own, it would not be easy taking her to the wound care center every Friday until she healed. Our assistant or I had to give her breakfast, bathe her, and dress her. Since she was about one hundred and thirty pounds of dead weight, Bill would often be the person who transferred her from the wheelchair, to the chair lift and held onto to her as chair came down the stairs. Then he transferred her back into the wheelchair and into the car. Once we arrived at the wound care center, Bill transferred her back into her wheelchair, pushed her up a ramp into the office, and transferred her onto the examination table. After she was done, all the work continued in reverse. I was so blessed to have Bill's help.

Getting her to wound care was not the worst of it. I always worried that one of the wounds would get infected beyond our control. With an older person, things can happen fast, without much warning. I thought I was ready for her passing. Honestly, I thought it might be a relief not to have to work so hard keeping my mother clean, fed, and well, but another part of me knew I would miss her very much.

Even though, my mother was no longer herself, no longer the person I once knew, I still could hug and kiss her and look into her big brown eyes. Once she was gone, I was sure the house and my heart would feel way too empty.

YOUR JOURNAL

What is in your mind and heart today?

TIP FOR CAREGIVER

Sometimes I didn't succeed, but I tried to go through my own refrigerator and my parents' often, getting rid of bowels and containers of food that were no longer good to eat. When I took the time to label leftovers with a cooked date, I didn't have to wonder how old something was.

Lullaby for Mother

Watch over my mother, Lord,
as you watch over the day.
When her thoughts were clear,
she trusted in your love
and your gift of grace.

Watch over my mother, Lord,
as I decide her care.
Please impart your wisdom
for choices I must make;
nothing's crystal clear.

Watch over my mother, Lord,
as you watch over a child.
She can't call your name
when she feels afraid,
but please stay by her side.

Watch over my mother, Lord.
Her time with me grows short.
It is your Holy choice
when she passes on,
becoming whole again.

I Thessalonians 5:16-18
"Be joyful always, pray at all times, be thankful in all circumstances. This is what God wants from you in your life in union with Christ Jesus."

The Grass is Greener

Too often I felt trapped taking care of my mother at home. Bill and I couldn't see our children and grandchild when we wanted. We couldn't go on vacation when we wanted. We couldn't sell our house and move south to get away from the snow in the winter as we wanted. Want. Want. Want. This is why I felt trapped because I wanted to be somewhere else or wanted to be doing something else.

Often I thought life would be so much easier if my mother were in a nursing home. Once again the old saying was mine; *the grass is always greener on the other side of the fence* or at least it seemed that way.

I still believed I could find peace though if I stopped concentrating on the all the fun Bill and I were missing. I had to remember that there were worse jobs in the world than taking care of my own dear mother who continued to have a sweet disposition. Peace would finally come to my soul if decided I was all right with this job, given to me by God.

YOUR JOURNAL

Have you ever felt like the grass is taller and sweeter on the other side of the fence?

TIP FOR CAREGIVER

We were paying big bucks for my mother's special bandages. One day a wound care nurse told us that Medicare should pay for them. She made a telephone call for us, and we got the bandages mailed to us at no cost. We wished we knew about this right from the beginning.

Gratitude

You know those big
orangey-red poppies
in our yard?
They're a favorite of mine.
Anytime I look
into their black insides
I say, *how beautiful.*
The same is true when I hear
a wren singing opera
in our apple tree.
But I thank God most
for you . . .
the multitude of colors
on our deck because you
planted flowers there
and the evening
when tired you leaned
into my parent's refrigerator
and cleaned the stubborn spills.

Romans 5:3-5

"We also boast of our troubles, because we know that trouble produces endurance, endurance brings God's approval, and his approval creates hope. This hope does not disappoint us, for God has poured out his love into our hearts by means of the Holy Spirit, who is God's gift to us."

Over and Over Again

My mother stopped having BMs once again. We realized Amitiza, the drug her gastroenterologist had given her, was not turning out to be the complete answer. Our assistant, Bill, and I worried as my mother's stomach got harder and more swollen. Her doctor and his associate made several recommendations of things we could try. Our assistant and I gave her the chemical used to prepare people for colonoscopies, but this did not work. We tried laxative suppositories using the "plug the dike method" with my latex gloved-finger holding it in place until it melted, but it did not work.

Several years ago, I had given my mother enemas. After that horribly messy and upsetting experience, I said I would never do it again, yet here I was giving her enemas out of desperation. Since it didn't work after a couple of times, I stopped, and then I worried that I quit too soon.

At some point, I asked the doctor if there was anything more he could do for my mother if we brought her to hospital, but he said no. He explained that she would either have a BM or die from impaction. His blunt words were shocking to here.

However, when all was said and done, the doctor did continue to help us. During these days of waiting, he added more and more chemicals to our arsenal of laxatives. Soon she was taking Amatiza, Miralax, and stool softener.

Our assistant had spoken to a nutritionist who said that perhaps the fiber was cutting down on mobility of the stool. At this point we were willing to try anything, so we stopped adding fiber to her drinks.

Maybe another enema helped or maybe moving her around one day as she went to several doctor appointments helped or perhaps the chemicals kicked in, but whatever the reason, my mother finally had a BM on the twelfth day. I was happy and thankful to God.

*

The pastor of our church was extremely supportive with her kind words of encouragement. She knew it had been difficult for Bill and me to take care of my parents and now just my mother. The following was part of an email I sent to her:

This morning, I think it has become clear to me that God is teaching me that the things I thought I couldn't or wouldn't do I can and will do. I said I wouldn't wipe George's bottom, but I had to. I said I'd never give my mother another enema, and here I am giving her several. I think God doesn't want me to be a chicken anymore. I am trying to be open to His teachings.

*

Our assistant and I continued to decrease and increase the chemicals we gave my mother. We worked toward an appropriate amount of prescription and non-prescription laxatives. Perhaps there was no such thing as just the right dose, but we monitored the situation closely. We certainly knew what could happen if she stopped going again. It was my constant fear.

YOUR JOURNAL

What is your secret fear regarding the health of your loved one?

TIP FOR CAREGIVER

When my parents moved to our house, they came with a supply of canned and boxed goods. Some appeared to be quite old since they did not have a nutritional facts panel, and others were bought at stores that were no longer in existence. Rather than wonder whether the food inside was still good, I dumped the stuff out. This made room for new items, and I did not have to worry that they might consume something that did not taste good or even worse yet made them sick.

January Thaw

I wipe a refrigerator spill,
wash out the bathroom,
plan supper.
The kitchen floor begs
for attention,
but my meniscus insists
it will wait another day.

Jack Frost took personal time,
allowing for rest on the deck.
My cells absorb sunshine,
soul food for a restless spirit.
Tranquility soothes tight tendons
until. . . I remember
Mom needs a trip to the ER
if the fourth laxative doesn't work.

Perhaps snow on the ground and
deer unable to find a blade of grass,
would have thrown me into
serious contemplation, but
today anxiety melts into puddles,
running toward an afternoon of perfection.

Psalm 86:3-5

"You are my God, so be merciful to me;
   I pray to you all day long.
Make your servant glad, O Lord,
   because my prayers go up to you.
You are good to us and forgiving,
   full of constant love for all who pray to you."

Change of Focus

Now we had another problem to worry about, Mom's persistent sores. She had two, one at the end of her spine and one on her buttocks. I was most concerned about the one that was the size of an apricot. Constantly I was reminded of this problem because it was my job to change the bandages daily. These bandages are made special so they do not need to be changed more than about twice a week, but my mother's wounds were located where her wet diaper loosened them.

I dreaded this job. First the wounds had to be washed with a mild soap and then rinsed. Paper towels were best for this purpose since they were more slippery than a washcloth and didn't drag against the wound. Next I used a sterile stick to apply two different kinds of suave on one of the wounds and only one kind on the other wound. Then I used a special wipe that helps the bandages stick to the skin. Lastly I applied the bandages, carefully so the sticky part did not touch the sore. I was exhausted from tension when I was through.

All these steps in changing the bandages were nothing compared to the sight and smell of the one larger wound. It made me upset just to look at it. Our assistant and I took such good care of my mother daily that it was shocking and sad that this had happened to her.

At church I requested that the minister include my mother in the prayers for those who had special needs. I also said my own prayers. Just as I had pleaded with God to let her have a BM, I begged Him now to heal her wounds.

Perhaps part of my desire for the wounds to go away was selfish since I hated to change those bandages. The hope that my mother would not suffer was mixed with my own wish that I would not have to deal with the sores anymore. Looking back I realize it was very human of me wanting to escape from this horrible job, but even then I knew God understood. God's forgiveness and His constant love were and still are a comfort to me.

YOUR JOURNAL

What is one of your reoccurring prayers for your loved one and yourself?

TIP FOR CAREGIVER

Some things in my parent's bathroom I cleaned quite often such as the toilet bowel and seat, the support rails on the walls near the toilet, and the sink. When I was organized, the rest of the bathroom, including the floor was a once a week job, unless an accident called for immediate attention.

After I washed the bathroom and it was shiny clean, I stood there and admired my work. It felt good to be finished, and it felt good to know this was another way I showed my love to God and my parents.

Holes

The cold air smells of linen
just off the clothesline, fresh and clean.
My boots crunch against the snow
as I avoid dark, ugly holes
left by those crazed, hotfooted bears
who came out of hibernation
for disco night under the stars.

The smile leaves my face when I remember,
I must change Mother's soggy bandage.
I dread the sight of that deep, oozing wound,
the color of a prune that smells like rotten meat.

Psalm 66:18-20

"If I had ignored my sins,
  the Lord would not have listened to me.
But God has indeed heard me;
  he has listened to my prayer.

I praise God,
  because he did not reject my prayer
or keep back his constant love from me."

Operation

When I changed Mom's bandage one evening, I noticed the area around one wound seemed extra red. The next morning I called the wound care center and was told to bring her into the office, but there might be a bit of a wait. Our caregiver and I scrambled to get my mother cleaned up, dressed, and out of the house as soon as possible.

I took the opportunity to stay home and get some housework done while our assistant and Bill took my mother to the wound care center. While they were gone, I scrubbed out our bathtub. Those self-cleaning bubbles were not enough for this sorely neglected tub. Then I swept and washed my mother's kitchen floor, taking the time to do an extra good job. As I worked I felt as if I was doing penance for not going with my mother to the wound care center. By the time they came home, the tub and floor were sparkling.

Not going with Mom did not shelter me from the bad news that came home with her. Mom needed same-day surgery in five days, and she had to have a pre-opt blood test. The doctor wanted to do a major cleaning of the wound, requiring a shot to numb the area and a sedative that could not be given at the office. I felt like someone had kicked me in the stomach even though I understood why it had to be done.

When we first brought her to the wound care center, the nurses and doctor explained that a wound does not heal with dead tissue present. In my mind, I understood the concept, but it has been difficult to watch the doctor scrape the wound, making it larger and larger every time she went for an appointment.

I knew the surgery would mean the wound would become even wider and deeper. Certainly my mother would be in lots of pain, and there was still no guarantee the wound would heal. We had been told due to my mother's weak circulatory system, it was hard for her body to heal.

I prayed God would be in charge and orchestrate everything. I prayed I would speak when necessary, and my mother would not suffer. At some point, I decided I had to stop repeating the prayer for no suffering. I had to trust God to answer this in the affirmative, so I began to thank Him. I felt like I was trying to manipulate God into action when I thanked Him in advance. Really though I knew He wanted to bless us with goodness. I would trust God to protect my mother from suffering.

Our assistant was off from work on the day my mother needed to have her pre-operative blood test. It was not easy getting her washed and dressed and fed as quickly as possible. I was sure my acid reflux would get me later, but in order for Mom to be on time, I rushed around like a mad woman with Bill's help.

Bill drove us to the hospital where we had been told to go for the blood test. We hauled my mother out of the car and into her wheelchair only to find out they had moved the lab to another location. Again Bill hauled my mother back into the car.

The lab was located only five minutes away from the hospital. It was a blessing that my mother was taken immediately, with no waiting. The lab technician made sure the proper insurance codes were in the computer and was able to take my mother's blood on the first try. God must have been with Mom because in the past many people had a terrible time drawing blood from her tiny veins that often collapsed. I was grateful that this time she didn't have to suffer more than one tiny prick. God is good.

YOUR JOURNAL

When was the last time you felt God protected you or your loved one?

TIP FOR CAREGIVER

Before George began renal dialysis, he was on an extremely strict diet that severely limited his protein intake. George was legally blind so would not know if I served my mother something else, but I didn't. Basically, I kept her on the same diet. Mistakenly, I thought that less meat in my mother's diet was a good thing, but apparently I had gone too far.

Maybe it was the diet or maybe it would have happened anyway but my mother got sick and ended up in the hospital with bronchitis. She also developed a wound that would not heal.

After her hospital stay, a nutritionist came to our home and explained that my mother needed more protein, vitamins, and minerals. These would promote good health and aid in the healing of her wound. Of course I immediately changed what I fed her for the better. Eventually, this first wound did go away.

Our assistant and I had learned from the nutritionists and doctors what my parents needed to eat for the best health possible. We also began to giving both my parents extra minerals and vitamins in pill form. Since my mother lost the ability to swallow pills, we crushed them and mixed it with a tablespoon of flavored yogurt, applesauce, jelly, or any food with a soft, moist consistency.

Plans

My plan was a watercolor masterpiece:
Chair in a Flower Garden, but
daffodils expanded into balloons,
crocuses ran into forsythias, and
the path washed away with the chair.

Another plan was to keep my mother
healthy until the end, but
now she is less the person
               and more the body
                            ravaged by sores.

Matthew 14:29-31

"'Come!' answered Jesus. So Peter got out of the boat and started walking on the water to Jesus. But when he noticed the strong wind, he was afraid and started to sink down in the water. 'Save me, Lord!' he cried.

At once Jesus reached out and grabbed hold of him and said, 'What little faith you have! Why did you doubt?'"

More of God's Guidance

I had prayed that God would orchestrate everything, regarding my mother's surgery. I also asked that God alert me if there was something I needed to do or say since I my mother could no longer make her own decisions.

Even though I said this prayer and wanted to trust God completely, the night before Mom's surgery, I was almost paralyzed with anxiety. The next day would be a difficult one. I went to bed at 7:30 PM, actually by accident because my brain was so muddled. I thought it was already 9 PM. When Bill informed me of the time, I didn't care. I just stayed in bed, thinking I needed rest; tomorrow was going to be horrible.

When I woke up, it was sometime between four and five AM. I began to visualize the scalpel going against my mother's wound, making it larger and causing her pain. The vision in my mind kept coming and coming. At the same time, something inside me said, *don't take her for the surgery; she's too old, too frail, she will not recover from this.*

I felt God was guiding me against this surgery. I wanted to listen and obey, but I knew I would need support in order to feel at peace about it. I asked God for signs that I had made the right decision.

The first sign came from my husband. He did not get annoyed when I woke him up early in the morning with the news that we would not take my mother for surgery. He was only slightly hesitant about my decision. He had voiced doubts in the past as to whether scraping the wound and making it bigger was a good thing. Now he repeated this same concern. We both understood the concept that dead tissue must be removed, but in my mother's case, we had not seen any improvement as the doctor cleaned it week after week in his office. Now that he wanted to do major scraping, both of us had no faith that this would be good for her.

Soon after I spoke with Bill, I called same-day-surgery to inform them I decided not to bring her in for the procedure. The lady who answered the telephone couldn't have been nicer. She said she understood, and she wished me good luck with my mother. To me this was yet another confirmation that I had made the right decision.

I called the pastor of our church and asked her to come to house for breakfast so we could pray together about my decision. When she arrived, she accepted that I was being led by God to cancel my mother's surgery. She also believed that it was possible that God had worked in my dreams, helping me to make this turn around as soon as I awoke. She said that this might be a good decision for now, but at some point things might change. I felt validated and supported by her words.

After the pastor left, my mother's friend called on the telephone, asking if my Mom had had the procedure. I told her I felt led by God not to bring her. She said that she had been praying that my mother would not have this surgery because she felt it would not be good for her. Well, I was nearly blown away. Again God was showing me that I had made the right decision.

Later in the day, I spoke with the doctor who would have done the surgery. He said that given my mother's advanced age, I made a reasonable decision. From now on he would not treat her wound aggressively, but only do what he had to do to prevent infection. He suggested that she come to wound care every two weeks instead of every week. Again, I felt God had led me to make the right decision.

Later I spoke on the telephone to my dear friend who lives a state away. She too agreed that God had guided me. Talking to her is always an uplifting experience. She always assures me that I have my mother's best interests in mind. When I do have selfish thoughts, she reminds me this is normal since I am human. Again her words supported me in my decision.

After a few hours passed, Bill said, *I believe you made the right decision.* His words were another wonderful blessing.

God had not left me alone. Again and again throughout the day He sent me messages through people around me, confirming that I made the right decision. He also gave me the strength to stand against Satan when doubts threatened my peace.

When night came, I slept soundly, and in the morning, I had peace about the decision I had made the day before. God is good.

*

A week later I still thanked God that He guided me in this direction. My mother had an appointment at the wound care center in a few days, and we would take it from there. Hopefully, the doctor would be able to keep her wound clean and free from infection.

YOUR JOURNAL

If you felt uneasy and unsure about a procedure your doctor suggested for your loved one, what steps would you take in the interest of making a wise decision?

TIP FOR CAREGIVER

When George was so tired that he refused to have a normal meal, we insisted he sit up for a few minutes to have one or two nutritional drinks. When my mother was about to miss a meal because of a doctor's appointment, we made sure we had one of these drinks and a straw with us.

In the interest of saving money, Bill shopped at the warehouse stores for my parents' high protein supplement drinks. Since George liked chocolate, and my mother liked vanilla, he always purchased a case of both and never allowed us to run out.

God's Providence

Now no one needs us back home, so
Bill and I hike with our grandson.
John runs ahead to the edge of a cliff.
My heart leaps into my throat
as he gazes at the river far below, but

my mother was the one who fell toward death.
Yet God caught her just in the nick of time,
letting her go only when it was her time.

Romans 8:18

"I consider that what we suffer at this present time cannot be compared at all with the glory that is going to be revealed to us."

Wrong Choice

Bill, our assistant, and I began to realize that I made a wrong decision by putting my mother under hospice care. These organizations are usually very good at making sure that people near death are comfortable in their remaining days or weeks, but the hospice in our area was not good for the care of my mother's wounds.

We had been renting my mother's hospital bed and an alternating-air mattress for a few years. The alternating-air mattress was necessary because of Mom's bedsores. It constantly changed the pressure on her skin, aiding in the circulation of blood to the wounds. The air mattress we rented seemed to be adequate for my mother's needs, was covered by Medicare, and we were satisfied.

Now that hospice was on board, they had to take over the rental of the hospital bed and alternating-air mattress, using their own vendor. Right away we noticed that the new mattress was thinner and more fragile. It did not appear to be as good as the one we had in the past. Now looking back, I wished we had rejected this inferior mattress right from the beginning.

During the two months my mother was under hospice care, this poorer quality mattress needed to be replaced four times because of leaks. The people at the office seemed helpless to get us a replacement right away. It always took three to four days until a new one came. This was extremely upsetting because the doctor at the wound care center said that my mother's wounds could get worse in just a few hours without an alternating-air mattress. Bill, our assistant, and I took turns calling the office, requesting immediate action from hospice, but to no avail.

The last time one of these mattresses failed, my mother did develop another bedsore. I became convinced hospice was making things worse for her rather than better. A short while later, I took my mother off this organization's care.

YOUR JOURNAL

What do you plan to do in the near future for some rest and relaxation?

TIP FOR CAREGIVER

Many senior ailments call for a low salt diet, and I discovered several good cookbooks for this purpose. I already knew that onion and garlic add flavor to otherwise bland food, but these cookbook recipes showed me how to add spices and herbs instead of salt.

Also, our caregiver and I tried to become informed about any adverse interactions between the foods my parents ate and the medications they took. One example: George was not supposed to have anything high in vitamin K since he was on a blood thinner. Vitamin K is given to patients who have taken an overdose of blood thinner and need their blood-clotting factor raised quickly.

Faith

I know the sun
        will never forget to shine.
I know the wren
        will never forget to sing.
I know my mother
        will never forget to love me.

Proverbs 17:17

"Friends always show their love. What are relatives for if not to share trouble?"

Proverbs 17:24

"An intelligent person aims at wise action, but a fool starts off in many directions."

A Big Mistake

    Two weeks after I had decided not to take my mother for major debridement of her wound, a large red lump appeared. I made a telephone call to the wound care center only to discover that her doctor was not in the office. The lady I spoke with told me that my only option was to wait until the next day for an appointment or take her to the ER.

    I dreaded the emergency room with a passion. Usually they performed tests on my mother that were unnecessary, and we waited hours for the results. Even if she was admitted into the hospital, there was a long wait until a bed was available.

    This time my reluctance to take my mother to the ER had life-threatening consequences. *I made a big mistake.* By four PM, I was forced to make a complete turnaround. Mom began to run a temperature of one hundred and three. First of all to my knowledge, my mother has never had such a high temperature, at least not under my watch, and secondly, I suspected that such a high temperature had to be extra dangerous for an elderly person.

    I called 911. An ambulance, a paramedic, and support volunteers were at our house within minutes. The paramedic told me that this temperature was indeed dangerous, so he suggested that I immediately give my mother an acetaminophen. It did bring down her temperature, but there were other more serious problems.

    By the time the ambulance arrived at the hospital, her blood pressure was beginning to drop. The kind and informative paramedic told me she was going into sepsis, a life threatening condition that happens when infection overwhelms a person's body.

Within minutes my husband joined us at the ER. I was glad to see him because this time I knew things were extremely serious; my mother might die. I was grateful to have Bill stand beside me as I made important decisions regarding my mother's care. *I love that man!*

At this time, my mother was still on hospice. This prompted the doctor to suggest that I might not want to treat this infection as aggressively as they would treat a much younger person. Aggressively meant an operation to install a port in her artery, the best delivery system for an antibiotic. Since my mother was already ninety and not in the best of physical condition anyway, I agreed this was not the way to go. I knew my mother didn't have much time left with us, and I didn't want her to suffer any more than she had to. Also I understood that if we treated this infection aggressively this time, it would not prevent her from getting another infection right away again. Her circulation was bad at this point, and there was a good chance that her wounds would never heal.

My mother was started on an on an intravenous antibiotic, and gradually her blood pressure began to rise. About midnight, she was taken by gurney down the hall, into an elevator and up to the fourth floor surgical unit. Since she had an open wound, I supposed this was the most logical place for her to be.

*

Since my mother still ran a low-grade fever a few days later, an infection control specialist was called in. I was pleased to see she was put on the same drug she had been on the last time she was in the hospital. This one had agreed with her system.

In the next few days, I tried to trust God and not worry. I was still nervous, since hard decisions might be ahead. If her wounds became a constant source of pain and infection, I may have to put a stop to treating her with antibiotics and let her go. I had to trust God and her doctor to guide me.

Many times through my life I had wished for siblings but perhaps never more than now. It would have been good to have a sister to share in my mother's care, especially now when decisions might become difficult. Then I reminded myself that God had provided me with good friends, a kind pastor, a supportive husband, and caring assistant who were always there for me when I needed them. Also I had a good friend, who lived far away, but she supported me over the telephone with her kind words and encouragement. I thanked God for all these people in my life.

YOUR JOURNAL

What character qualities do you appreciate in your closest confidant?

TIP FOR CAREGIVER

In the last year of George's life, his appetite became almost nonexistent. Our assistant and I made him lots of soup that went down his throat easier than solids. We packed the soup with small pieces of meat and vegetables, providing excellent nutrition. My mother also enjoyed this type of meal, but we would puree hers since she no longer could use her dentures.

God' Work

Driving home from the hospital,
the moon plays hide-and-seek
behind dark tree trunks.
When I reach the top of the driveway,
its portly face seems to lounge
on our roof
like an upright dinner plate.
My empty stomach grumbles.

Supper will taste good tonight
now that my conscience is clear.
Mother's doctor agreed with me;
less aggressive treatment
is the right decision.
See, God did guide me after all.

I maneuver the car near the garage
where temperamental floodlights
decide to be agreeable.
They beam brightly in a wide arc.
After I park the car,
I run into the house, shivering.
It's way too cold for mid-March.

Before my jacket is off,
the aroma of spice and herbs is proof of love.
*Your friends called,
asking about you and your mother*, he says.
I smile and sit at the table, allowing myself
a full portion of gratitude.
It is good when we all do God's work.

James 1:2-3

"My friends, consider yourselves fortunate when all kinds of trials come your way, for you know that when your faith succeeds in facing such trials, the result is the ability to endure."

More Guidance

I sat in my mother's hospital room, watching her intently. Again I prayed God would help me to somehow know that I had made the right decision. I was tortured by doubt because I had not allowed aggressive treatment of Mom's wounds, yet I knew at her age and given her extremely bad circulation, there were no guarantees that the surgery would have bought her much more time. So far, this was the hardest decision I had ever made. I believed that God had guided me against the procedure, but I needed His reassurance once again.

God answered my prayer with the words of two of my mother's doctors. The first doctor I spoke with specializes in infection control, and he determined the appropriate intravenous antibiotic for my mother. I asked him if he agreed with me, not to treat my mother's wound aggressively. He said, *it* was *a reasonable* decision. (Later I looked up this word in the dictionary. It means *possessing sound judgment.*)

The second doctor I spoke with was her wound care doctor. I hoped he would say more than the word *reasonable*; I needed more. After I asked him to be honest with me, he said that given the fact she was elderly and had other medical issues, he would not want to treat her wounds aggressively. *Phew!* I so much needed to hear him say just those words.

As I sat in a chair next to my mother's bed and fed her, I saw an innocent helpless look on her face. This was the face I loved and the same face that all my life meant strength and comfort. It was difficult to know that my decision might take her away sooner rather than later, yet I believed God had brought me to that decision. He still would continue to guide me to do His will for my mother.

It seemed like a paradox: I believed that my decision might take my mother from this life. At the same time, I believed that only God decides when we die. How could both be true? Whether right or wrong both concepts seemed to exist inside me side-by-side. Maybe when God makes the decision to take us home, He somehow uses human decisions to implement His will. *Who knows?* This is one of the mysteries of life.

Bill picked me up early from the hospital because a Nor'easter was beginning to bury all the roads in our area with cold white stuff. It was hard to leave my mother's bedside, knowing someone else would give her supper. I was sure they would not cut up her food as fine as she needed, but I hoped they would at the very least give her the nutrition drink that comes with the meal.

I loved my mother so very much. At this point, she was helpless, and it broke my heart to leave her at the hospital with people who did not understand her like I did. I prayed: *Please God take care of my mother. Watch over her and protect her.*

*

The next day Bill and I were knee-deep in snow as we shoveled and snow-blew our way out of the driveway. Our goal was to get me to the hospital as soon as possible. Then my mother would finally have a good meal through my diligent effort.

YOUR JOURNAL

When someone else takes care of your loved one, do you ever worry they won't do as good a job as you?

TIP FOR CAREGIVER

Often I felt trapped by all the responsibility that came with the care of my parents at home, but one thing always helped me greatly, my crockery pot. The morning has always been my energy time, so preparing foods to go into the crock-pot early in the day was easy for me. Then I felt good, knowing our meal would we ready on time for supper.

Here and There

Here our feet are almost frozen,
our backs begin to break, and
we long for summer while
we shovel out the driveway.
Last night winds and clouds
whelped a heavy, white beast
who refuses to budge without a fight.

There Mother is warm and comfortable
in a big, white bed, but
she needs our hugs and kisses.
She smiles at angels with nametags
who try to feed her, but
they fly away before she's done.

No magic vanquishes the white beast
who seems bigger-by-the-minute, but
God's protection remains here and there.

Nahum 1:7

"The Lord is good;
  he protects his people in times of trouble;
  he takes care of those who turn to him."

Blood Transfusion

Soon again, God guided me to make another important decision for my mother. At some point during her stay at the hospital, the doctor called me at home with the news that Mom's hemoglobin was low which could cause her shortness of breath and loss of appetite. The most aggressive way to treat this condition would be to give her two units of blood. He also offered the less aggressive and slower acting treatment of giving her iron. Since my mother was already having a hard time eating. I asked him if the transfusion would be painful, and he said it would not. To me this transfusion would be a decision to keep my mother comfortable. My thinking was that anything that made her feel better and did not cause pain was a good thing. With the help of a nurse, the doctor and I did a telephone-consent.

It was interesting to me that I opted not to treat Mom's wounds aggressively, but I let her have a blood transfusion. Of course, the operation on my mother's wounds would have caused pain, and there was a good chance it would not have cured them. The blood transfusion would not hurt her and might do her some good. I believed that God wanted me to use my common sense and also count on His guidance.

I wondered if soon another hard decision would come my way. Again, my mother ran a low-grade temperature. It puzzled me that after a week of antibiotics that that this still would happen. If intravenous antibiotics must be continued longer than the usual seven to ten days, I knew she might run out of good veins. In fact, while I was visiting my mother at the hospital, the technician that changed the intravenous site and expressed the same concern. She wanted to know if I ever thought about a port in my mother's artery for this purpose. I told her that since I had opted for non-aggressive treatment, I hoped this procedure could be avoided.

*

It was early morning, and I was at home. I wondered if the doctor would call me later to express his concern about the low-grade temperature. Could it be that her body was unable to overcome this infection even with the huge dose of antibiotics she had already received? I had thought she was out of danger for the time being and on her way home. Now I was not so sure.

YOUR JOURNAL

What steps do you take when you must make a hard decision for yourself or your loved one?

TIP FOR CAREGIVER

There was a time when our assistant and I had the goal of serving meals to my stepfather and mother at the kitchen table. George would use his cane and later, a walker, but it was easy for him to get to his seat. At first my mother could walk to her chair, but later she sat close to the table in her wheelchair.

In time, things changed. George got more tired, and so did we. It seemed easier to bring the food into the living room and put it on a tray in front of his lift chair. Our assistant or I sat in a chair near my mother's lift chair to help her eat. We all were entertained since there was a television in this room.

God's Guidance

Lucy sneaks on Ricky's show;
the pig runs wild on *Green Acres*;
Guy conducts old time music;
our gang hides from the truant officer.

Then it was easy to watch television with
a woman who thought rain on the screen
meant it was raining outside.

Now things are different.
My decisions for her have become life or death.
We are lost in a medical world where
rules can be wrong, and
nothing is reliable except God's guidance.

Psalm 37:23-24

"The Lord guides us in the way we should go
  and protects those who please him.
If they fall, they will not stay down,
  because the Lord will help them up."

Doubts and Fears

To be perfectly honest, at this point, I was afraid to bring my mother home from the hospital. Just the thought of changing her bandages again upset me. Her bedsores were horrendous to look at, and at times the odor was appalling. No matter how hard our assistant and I tried to give her good care, the sores would not heal. Also they had become infected, and now we knew how easily this could kill her.

The thought of her coming home with the urinary tract catheter that had been put in place at the hospital was also upsetting since it would add another unpleasant job and worry. The thing had to be emptied often and sometimes the bag needed to be replaced. Also the catheter made her highly susceptible to a urinary tract infection. No wonder I was afraid to bring my mother home.

If I choose to be optimistic, I would tell myself that I would get used to changing her bandages again and dealing with the catheter. If her wounds became infected, this time I would act quickly to get her the right medication. Our assistant and I would continue to give my mother lots of cranberry juice to ward off a urinary tract infection. I had to admit though, I was tired of all this and wished someone else would take care of my mother.

Once again, I considered a nursing home, and once again, Bill warned me that she probably would not get the kind of good care she was getting at home. He reminded me that these homes on occasion do not have enough people on staff. This meant there was a real possibility that my mother might be neglected from time to time. Well, that was the end of that idea, although it was a strong temptation.

If only my mother didn't have horrible wounds, she would be relatively easy to take care of, and her health would be so much better. The severity of these wounds made me think that she might die soon. We already knew from a test that my mother's circulation was extremely bad in her legs, but now the wound care doctor told me that this problem could be in her torso as well, and perhaps this was the reason she was not healing from the wounds at the bottom of her spine. Probably this was why she had developed two new wounds in the past two weeks.

I had to prepare myself that my mother may be dying soon. If I did not stand in God's way, I hoped He would prevent my mother from suffering and take her to heaven. I continued to pray for His guidance.

YOUR JOURNAL

Do believe God always has the final word when someone will die?

TIP FOR CAREGIVER

When my mother could use a cup, I would place a heavy towel across her chest in case of major spills. At some point she started to have difficulty lifting a coffee mug to her mouth. We were not sure why this occurred, but we theorized her arthritis and her increased dementia had something to do with it. We did not give up on her; instead, I bought her a bunch of colorful plastic mugs. They turned out to be a good solution for all her liquids. They were lightweight, and the larger handles were easier for her to grab. These cups also decreased the number of accidental spills.

Eventually the spills came so often that our assistant and I realized she was too weak and too confused to hold even a light plastic mug. We discovered that it was easier for her to sip liquid through a straw as one of us held the drink in front of her.

At Last Light

At dusk I stand nearby,
watching the birds take
their final trips to the feeder.
Mom's prognosis whispers
louder out here
among long shadows while
lingering rays
paint the sky tangerine.

I ask the chickadee,
How did this happen while
she was in my care?
He takes a seed and flies away,
leaving no answer.
I ask the wren,
Does God appoint our time to die?
She too takes a seed and
flies away in silence.

An impatient gust of wind,
chills my neck, and
I choose God's wisdom as
the last light begins
to sink out of sight.

Psalm 73:25-26

"What else do I have in heaven but you?
   Since I have you, what else could I want on earth?
My mind and my body may grow weak,
   but God is my strength;
   he is all I ever need."

Money Matters

When my mother's doctor said my mother needed a blood transfusion, because her hemoglobin was low, he told me that since she was under hospice care, it made it difficult for him to order a transfusion. By this time, I had already taken my mother off this service, but as yet, I had not informed her doctor.

A few months later, the reason the doctor hesitated about the transfusion hit Bill and I right between the eyes. The date my mother came off hospice became extremely important as to who would pay her huge hospital bills. We came to find out that if a person is on this service, life-extending treatment is not covered. The thinking being that the person is likely to die soon with or without further treatment.

Since no one had explained this to me, it was a good thing that I had taken my mother off hospice at the beginning of her hospital stay. Otherwise, the transfusion and perhaps some other hospital bills would not have been covered by Medicare. This taught us a huge lesson.

Hospice is an excellent organization for short-term comfort and support for the dying and their family, but now we understood not to call in this service until our loved-one was near death and did not need any more procedures, tests or specialists.

YOUR JOURNAL

Write out your thoughts on end of life care. You may want to check if your loved one has a will, living will, and health care proxy documents in place.

TIP FOR CAREGIVER

When George's fluid intake had to be monitored closely, our assistant and I poured the allotted amount of water into a container and refrigerated it. If we gave him pills or made his oatmeal, we poured from this container. When he had an eight-ounce glass of cranberry juice each day, we subtracted this amount of fluid from the container.

In the Jungle of Life

where deadly fangs and claws
lurk behind thick bushes,

we reach our destination,
not knowing how many times
You saved us from calamity.

Psalm 69:1-3

"Save me, O God!
   The water is up to my neck;
I am sinking in deep mud,
   and there is no solid ground;
I am out in deep water,
   and the waves are about to drown me.
I am worn out from calling for help,
   and my throat is aching.
I have strained my eyes,
   looking for your help."

Today

I was anxious and had a heavy heart. My mother's condition was worse and harder to deal with. Yesterday, when the phlebotomist tried to change the intravenous sight, she could not find a good vein on my Mom's body. A technician telephoned me to ask if I would allow a pick line to be inserted into a larger vein. She made me feel it was a comfort decision since Mom would never have to be pricked again. She said the pick could stay in a whole year. Since this would mean less pain for my mother, I gave my permission.

Later that same day when I arrived at the hospital, I wasn't so sure I had made the right decision. The lady I spoke with over the telephone had failed to inform me that this pick would need careful attention each day to prevent clotting and infection. When I took Mom home from the hospital this pick would be another worry. Already she had four wounds that had to be cleaned and bandaged on a regular basis. Also the urinary tract catheter bag needed daily attention. And now I would need to empty two syringes of fluid into each one of the two access tubes on her pick line. I felt overwhelmed and scared.

When I came from the hospital, I was more upset than I had been in a very long, long time. Many thoughts were going through my mind. *I can't do this; that's why I decided not to become a nurse. I can force myself, but I don't want to. I want the best for my mother, so I must force myself to deal with this.* Bill and our assistant both said they would do the *syringe part for me, but I don't want to wash my mother's bottom anymore either. I don't want to see those wounds any more when I change the bandages. It is not fair to Bill that he must do the syringes even if he is willing. I don't think my mother will last very long anyway. It appears her days are numbered. Am I not accepting God's strength to continue taking care of her or does God want me to put her in a nursing home at this point? Maybe God is saying, "You don't have to take care of her anymore."*

YOUR JOURNAL

Do you have a limit for what you will do for a loved one?

TIP FOR CAREGIVER

When my stepfather's fluids were restricted, fluids were what he wanted most. This was emotionally difficult for him and us. It was upsetting for him to hear, *No, it's too soon for another cup of water.* He told us he had to have water with his meals or else the food wouldn't go down, so we started to let him have most of his fluids when he ate, and he was only given a swallow with his pills. Sometimes he would need one sip in between meals, just to wet his whistle.

Blocks

While I slept, a monster loaded
cement blocks onto my chest.
I awoke gasping for air.

Overnight my mother's medical care
became more difficult, making me feel
like a child asked to do surgery.

I will not move from this spot
until a grownup lifts these blocks away.

Psalm 94:18-19

"I said, 'I am falling';
  but your constant love, O Lord, held me up.
Whenever I am anxious and worried,
  you comfort me and make me glad.."

Yes or No?

I had to make a decision right away. I prayed for clear guidance what to do. Unless God changed my mind, I was once again leaning toward a nursing home for my mother. I prayed God would make sure she went to a good one and would continue to protect her. There are many nursing homes in our area, and I did not know which one would be just right for her. I would trust God to guide me.

Even though I asked God for His help, I also believed I had to do my part. I telephoned two of my girlfriends who have had mothers in two different nursing homes in the area. Both of them were pleased and had no compliments.

With the names of these nursing homes in hand, Bill and I met with a case manager at the hospital. I told her that I had been wishing someone would say to me that I don't have to take care of my mother anymore. Immediately, she said the words I wanted to hear. *You don't have to take care of your mother anymore.* She was a kind lady. She said she would call the two homes to see if they had a bed for my mother. I felt relieved, but at the same time this would be a big change. I was also scared and still wondered if this was the right move for my mother and me.

Shortly after we met with the case manager, God showed me He had other plans. I had prayed for Him to orchestrate everything and change my mind if necessary. God already knew what was about to happen.

Our assistant did not want my mother to go to a nursing home unless that was truly what I wanted. She volunteered to take on the job of attending to my mother's pick, urinary catheter, and wounds if we decided to bring her home. Bill added that he also would learn how to do these things for Mom for the times our assistant was not available. I was pleasantly surprised. Now I would not have to put my mother in a nursing home. Now I could breathe again, and if my mother did come out of the hospital, she would come back home.

*

After the pick line was inserted and my mother was back in her hospital bed, she fell asleep so soundly that I couldn't feed her supper. From now on, Bill, our assistant, and I found it difficult getting Mom eat and drink anything. Every time I couldn't feed her I became upset and discouraged because I knew what would happen if this continued.

She would eventually die without the proper nutrition and hydration, but I had already turned down the option of a feeding tube inserted into her stomach. Doctors I spoke with and a book I was given about end of life issues both agreed, putting a patients with end stage dementia on a feeding tube usually was not successful. In these cases, the g-tube caused other life-threatening problems.

Even though I believed that Mom would have understood that I was trying to make the best decision under the circumstances, I still felt guilty. I loved her and wondered how I could just stand by and let her die, but I also did not want her to suffer any more than necessary.

It also occurred to me that if I allowed a feeding tube that I might get in God's way if He planned to take her to heaven. This was probably a silly thought because God is all-powerful, and He will always do what is the very best for each one of His children. Since I prayed that God would orchestrate everything, I trusted that His will would be done. He was in control.

Even though I knew God was with me and would guide me every step of the way, again I felt too alone being an only child. It would be such a comfort if my sibling agreed or disagreed with me about the feeding tube. An agreement would bring me a sense of peace, and a disagreement would make me rethink what I thought was best after all. Either way it would be a help to discuss Mom's care with someone who loved her as much as I did.

Once again, I reminded myself that God had placed good and caring people by my side. Also, He had provided me with everything I needed all these nine years as I took care of my parents. He would continue to guide me, and watch over my mother.

YOUR JOURNAL

Do you have the support of someone who cares for your loved one as much as you do?

TIP FOR CAREGIVER

Every time George went to dialysis, he took a vinyl bag we filled with a non-leak plastic container of water, a soft pillow for him to sit on, and a lap blanket. All of these items were essential to his comfort during a long and cold dialysis session.

Since George was legally blind, it was hard for him to deal with a vinyl bag that completely collapsed every time he placed it on the floor. I cut up a sheet of plastic canvas that I got from the craft store and made a frame for the inside of his bag to keep it stiff and open.

Lost

My husband and I hike
among pines that
refuse to point out the shortest way.
Trudging through mud and rock,
we follow a brook uphill,
Our sneakers slip, our ankles wobble,
and we lose our way for an hour.

Later at the hospital,
I ponder whether to relinquish
Mom's care to strangers.
It is then I realize I am still lost.

Matthew 7:1-2

"Do not judge others, so that God will not judge you, for God will judge you in the same way you judge others, and he will apply to you the same rules you apply to others."

Now I Understand

My mother began to run a temperature of over 100 degrees, and her skin was bright red. The same infection control doctor who had been on her case in the past was called in. This pleased me since I trusted him. He looked at all four of her wounds and said they were not infected, but he felt she did have a rash. He thought that perhaps she might be having an allergic reaction. He stopped all of her medication. He ordered some tests and told me we might know more later.

I continued to trust that God was in control. This thought continued to give me a sense of peace and comfort.

*

I spent the whole day with my mother from morning till night. One of the many times that I said, *I love you*, I thought Mom mumbled the same words back to me. She ate quite well the day before, and this day she appeared stronger.

Day by day, there had been new challenges for me to deal with. Sometimes Mom seemed better and the next she was not. I tried to prepare myself for whatever might be coming, if that were even possible

*

I found it interesting that I got so very close to putting my mother in a nursing home. One of the homes had already sent someone to see my mother. She determined that my mother would be a good match with the lady who would become her roommate.

Maybe God wanted me to understand from a personal point of view how hard it is to relinquish control and care of a parent to a nursing home. I found it frightening. Now I understood, not only how emotionally and physically draining it can be to take care of a parent at home, but I also understood that there is a sense of guilt when a nursing home becomes necessary. This guilt arises because the caregiver knows his or her parent will no longer enjoy the one-on-one care and attention given at home. Making it worse, often this decision must be made in a hurry with little time to find just the right place, one that is clean, well-staffed, and has a good reputation.

When Bill and I were considering this option, the case manager had explained that the beauty of a place is not important, but *the nurse to patient ratio* is key as to whether good care is provided. My concern was how often they would change Mom's diaper and how much time they would spend feeding her when I wasn't there. Even if the nursing home seemed like the very best, I had already decided that I would need to be an alert advocate for my mother, making sure all continued to go well.

Hopefully, there are many good nursing homes out there that do the best for their population. Unfortunately there are always those that do not have enough staff, and the people in their care suffer the consequences. I wish our state and federal government would pass stronger regulations for nursing homes and hire more inspectors to make sure these regulations are being met.

*

If I didn't have God on my side, I was sure I would feel completely lost. There had been so many big and scary decisions to make recently, and my mother was old and frail. *God will orchestrate everything*, I continued to remind myself. I don't know why this particular mantra was in my head constantly, but it never failed to give me peace.

YOUR JOURNAL

Write out a Bible verse or an uplifting sentence that can encourage you when things get difficult and scary. Memorize it.

TIP FOR CAREGIVER

I feel so fortunate that our assistant and I were able to rise above any silly misunderstandings that were sometimes unavoidable as she helped me take care of my parents. She turned out to be exactly the person I needed, and I do believe God sent her right to our door. Even now after my parents have passed away, we are still friends.

Our assistant's greatest qualification turned out to be her devotion to her own mother. Years before she applied for this job, she faithfully took care of her mother who had to be in a full-body cast after a fall. This wasn't an easy undertaking since, at the time, our assistant also had young children, including an infant to care for. After I heard this, I knew she had a good heart, and this turned out to be true.

Looking back I realize that I should have asked for references before hiring anyone. Also, I should have made up a list of daily chores we both signed. I thank God he gave me the insight I needed to hire the right person even if I foolishly didn't do my homework.

The Great Composer

Our Great Composer raises his baton
We in the orchestra pit hold our breath and wait.
None of us know how fast or how slow the notes will go.
It is He who understands the music.
It is He who leads us through each measure.

John 14:15-16

"If you love me, you will obey my commandments. I will ask the Father, and he will give you another Helper, who will stay with you forever."

Home Cancelled

Yesterday, my mother's doctor signed the paper to discharge my mother from the hospital. He called our home early in the morning to inform me of his decision.

Since the weekend was almost upon us, right away I went into overdrive. I had to find out from the case manager where we could get the supplies we needed for maintenance of my mother's port, the catheter, and the wounds. I knew she already had been alerted that we would need the services of a nurse affiliated with a home care agency in our area. This nurse would come to the home and open the case within twenty-four hours and continue to provide the necessary supplies for Mom's health needs. Despite that I felt I needed to be sure we had the right supplies ahead of time since the nurse probably wouldn't come to our house until Monday.

The case manager was not at her desk. I had to leave a message that included all my concerns and a request for her to call for an ambulance to transport Mom home. A nurse had suggested to me that this was necessary since my mother had stage four wounds.

Our assistant had a doctor's appointment, so I was the one who would go to the hospital and wait for the ambulance. God must have known I was needed there. As soon as I arrived, I was informed that the doctor ordered my mother's port taken out. I was extremely puzzled by this. Someone from the radiology department had explained to me that it could stay in place up to a year. After speaking with Mom's general doctor over the telephone, I realized I had been led astray. The doctor explained that no one is sent home with a port unless the person must continue to receive intravenous medication.

It troubled me that I had been misled. This prompted me to speak with a patient advocate, telling her that I might have made a different decision if I knew this new information. She told me that she would pass on my complaint to the radiology department. Later I did speak to someone from this department. I suggested it be made clear the port usually comes out when the patient goes home. Obviously it was too late for my mother, but hopefully others would benefit from my words.

Right after I spoke with my mother's general doctor, the infection control doctor appeared right in front of me, another sign that I was supposed to be there on this morning. This same doctor a few days earlier stopped giving my mother an antibiotic when she had another bad reaction. He had said that he might send her home on an oral antibiotic. I wanted to know if this was still his plan. He explained she was infection free and had decided against it. I didn't question him any further, but I thought perhaps her recent bad reactions to antibiotics might have changed his mind as well.

Before I spoke with the nurse on duty, I went in to see my mother. At that time my eyes focused on her swollen arm and hand. It was something we have seen before due to arthritis, but now it seemed more swollen. It looked like her skin could break open because of the pressure.

When the nurse saw it, she called the radiology department. After someone from that department checked my mother, it was suggested that Mom's doctor order a sonogram of her arm and shoulder. She informed me that these ports often form a blood clot. The nurse called the doctor and the test was ordered. Then I was informed that Mom's ride home in the ambulance would be put on a delay until the test was done.

Our assistant relieved me at around twelve-thirty pm, and I gladly took a break away from the hospital. I felt extremely shaken and needed to relax.

Later, after I got home, our assistant called me to say my mother would not be coming home. She did have a clot in her shoulder and would need to receive heparin, a clot-busting medication. This new problem had seemed to come out of nowhere, and I felt like I was being pulled apart and worn down.

All night I was restless, but in the morning things did improve. Our assistant went to the hospital early and called me with the news that my mother was receiving heparin, and her arm and hand were not as swollen as the day before. Now I felt relieved, but still nervous at the same time. When Mom came home, she'd be in a fragile state. At least good people were helping me, and I praised God for his guidance.

YOUR JOURNAL

What are your worries and concerns today?

TIP FOR CAREGIVER

Our assistant had many jobs to do, but as time went on, I realized which ones were important to me. One or both of my parents needed help with bathing and brushing their teeth, getting dressed, eating, and taking medications. Sometimes the bathroom needed a quick cleanup. Often meal planning and preparation were needed, especially if Bill and I were away. Along with that went the job of keeping the kitchen and eating surfaces neat and clean. Then there was always the laundry.

There was another thing that was not a job but was certainly important to me. If at all possible I wanted notice of at least twenty-four hours when our assistant couldn't come to work. Of course, emergencies might happen and certainly I tried to be flexible in those cases.

Because I counted our assistant as a friend, I always offered to listen and help her in any way I could when she was going through a particularly hard time in her life. We all have moments when we need someone to listen, not only with ears but also with a kind heart. She always did the same for me.

An Open, Wider Door

We wait for a crowded train.
Certainly I am not to blame.
Our bags are packed and
at the station.
Why, oh why, this hesitation?
Is this right or wrong, dear me?
God wants what's best, you see.
The train comes; we turn away.
We're not allowed on board today.

We'll go home; we'll pray some more.
God will show us what's in store
through an open wider door.

John 14:27

"Peace is what I leave with you; it is my own peace that I give you. I do not give it as the world does. Do not be worried and upset; do not be afraid."

Rollercoaster

My mother's stay in the hospital had been like a rollercoaster ride, zooming upward when the antibiotics worked, plummeting down when there was an allergic reaction, up when she ate a good meal, down when she was too tired to swallow liquids, up when she tried to talk with visitors, down when she needed a transfusion, up when she said I love you, down when she formed a blood clot in her arm.

I was not sure how my mother felt about all of this because she accepted what happened like an infant. She did not seem to be afraid or in pain. My prayers had always been for my mother not to suffer. Praise God; He had answered me in the affirmative on this one.

The rollercoaster ride took its toll on my nervous system, though. Rather than completely resting in the assurance that God was in charge, many times I allowed myself to become agitated. When this happened my body to went into the "flight or fight" mode. Then I was in overdrive, feeling out of control, not trusting God to do His part.

I prayed that God would orchestrate my mother's care, that doctors, nurses, techs, and lab people would have extreme wisdom in dealing with my mother. I also prayed I would speak when necessary as an effective advocate.

Since God is faithful, He was covering every part of my mother's care. I needed to relax. My trust and confidence in God would keep me sane and allow me the energy to take care of Mom.

I understood my mother might die soon, and the conscious part of me seemed to accept this, but who knew what was going on in my subconscious? There I suspected I was still the helpless child, screaming for her mommy not to leave. I reassured myself, *You're a big girl now; you'll be all right without your mother.* However, there was no way to know if I could prepare myself for her death.

Mom always made me feel loved, always made me feel special, and always forgave me when I was bad. Dementia had taken her away from me already. For many years now, I missed her friendship, but after she passed from this earth, I would miss the hugs and kisses I gave her and her big, beautiful brown eyes.

YOUR JOURNAL

What do you love most about the person you care for?

TIP FOR CAREGIVER

I grew to understand that I needed to be more flexible in the interest of keeping a good working relationship and friendship going with our assistant. Soon I realized as my parents became weaker, she had more work to do, which meant some things had to slide. Even my mother's sister told me as long as our assistant was good to my parents, I shouldn't worry about her not doing housework.

Of course, I did continue to voice my suggestions since I felt an open communication was the only way to go. However, there were times I was just plain petty, insisting on things that weren't all that important. Also I am sorry for my recommendations and reminders that came down too hard or at the wrong time.

Looking back, I am grateful that our assistant stuck with us anyway. She kept my parents safe, comfortable, and happy. She saved Bill and me from despair. She was and still is one of my best friends.

Cataclysmic Thoughts

I lay here in the cool, quiet dark.
No celestial lanterns shine through the curtains.
A gnawing sensation in my chest
will not let me rest, as if by some fluke
the safety of the planet is in my hands.

Watching my mother die is to know
the sun, moon, and stars will all go out.
There will be no more salty ocean breezes,
fragrant cut grass, and sweet spring flowers.

Next to me he sleeps soundly,
without knowledge
of my cataclysmic thoughts.

I get out of bed, rush for the thermostat, and
head for the kitchen where
for the time being, prayer and coffee will
return everything back where it belongs.

James 1:2-3

"My friends, consider yourselves fortunate when all kinds of trials come your way, for you know that when your faith succeeds in facing such trials, the result is the ability to endure."

Tired

My mother had been in the hospital for almost three weeks. Thankfully my prayers had been answered in the affirmative. My mother did not appear to be uncomfortable or in any pain. Even though I knew God was on our side, from a purely selfish point of view, I wanted freedom from my responsibilities as a caregiver. I was soul tired. My enthusiasm for life was plummeting.

Earlier in the day when I had more energy, I had decided to cook supper, but on the way home from the hospital, I already knew it was not going to happen. This troubled me since Bill and I had been eating out far too many times recently, not a healthy situation.

It was almost 5 PM when I got home. Bill was in another county playing racket ball, but I knew he'd call me before his trip home. It was then I asked him to pick up some take-out food. He was glad to do it. During this stressful period in my life, I was blessed by God to have a supportive and caring husband. Without his help, I would have had to give up on being a home caregiver a long time ago.

I woke up at five-thirty AM, a usual occurrence since my mother had been in the hospital. A barrage of disturbing thoughts about Mom's condition sent me catapulting out of bed. Immediately, I wrote the list of all my concerns and called her nurse at the hospital, asking her to pass on the list to Mom's doctor.

My message included five questions: Why were my mother's arms jerking around? Why was she more lethargic recently? Was the wound on her leg worse? What were the red botches on her arm? Why was her leg swollen? The nurse was kind and gladly took down everything I said.

*

My mother's assistant was at the hospital early, so I thought perhaps the doctor would address my concerns with her, but then again he might call me. From past experience, he seemed to resist staying in touch. I understood he was busy, but I needed to know that my mother was getting the best care possible. I was not looking for miracles, but I did want the doctor to be alert when he came to see her. Hopefully nothing important would be overlooked.

YOUR JOURNAL

What list of qualities should a good doctor have?

TIP FOR CAREGIVER

My parents had been in the hospital many times, and I always had the same concern. How could I encourage good communication with the doctor? Looking back, maybe I could have made things much easier for myself if I spoke with him on the first day of each hospital stay. I could have asked him if he was willing to call me with updates that would keep me informed of any changes.

Soul Tired

I wake up to wheels grinding to a crawl.
   What's wrong?
   What's right?
   What matters?
   What doesn't?
The energy flow is down to a trickle,
and there is no clear solution
how to fix it.

Psalm 92:1-2

"How good it is to give thanks to you, O Lord,
  to sing in your honor, O Most High God,
to proclaim your constant love every morning
  and your faithfulness every night . . ."

Waiting for X-Ray Results

Our assistant was off which meant I was the one at the hospital most of the day. I noticed that every time my mother took a breath, there was a gurgling sound. Also, I could not get her to wake up. The doctor was talking about sending her home, but I just did not think he understood her condition. I told him that if I took her home now she would die because I would not be able to get liquids or food into her. He ordered an x-ray of her lungs, but it was the weekend and everything progressed slowly. It wasn't until mid-afternoon that they finally took the x-ray. This meant I had to go home without knowing the results.

*

When I woke up around 3 AM, I called my mother's nurse, but the x-ray results still had not come in. I felt sick at heart; I worried that her condition might be getting worse. Then Bill reminded me that God was in charge. I agreed, but I worried that someone's misguided freewill might get in the way. I had been praying for God's will, but if someone's negligence caused my mother's death, then how could I count on this being God's will? I knew that a question like this was useless to contemplate because there would never be an answer.

It was clear to me though that I could always trust God. I had asked Him to orchestrate my mother's care, and I believed He had done just that. Now she seemed closer to death, I could not allow myself to think God had stopped watching over her. He was in charge. If He wanted her to live, she would. If He wanted her to die, she would. It occurred to me that if God took Mom to heaven, perhaps this was His way to protect her from pain and suffering. Her body had wounds that would not heal. If she lived, the road ahead could be one infection after another, not to mention pneumonia from her swallowing problems.

What Bill had said to me was true, God was in charge. God is faithful. God never fails. This truth was where I found peace.

YOUR JOURNAL

When your sense of peace is threatened, what do you tell yourself?

TIP FOR CAREGIVER

Anytime I visited my mother or stepfather in the hospital, I always brought along a canvas bag of things to keep myself entertained when they were sleeping or watching television. This gave me an opportunity to catch up on my crocheting, reading, or writing. It also helped my mind and body to stay relaxed.

Often I would bring lunch, a drink, or a snack. This saved money, and I continued to eat healthy foods. It seems strange to me that a place dedicated to making people well serves high fat food in their cafeteria. In their defense, they did offer many low-fat items as well, but the macaroni and cheese and the greasy hamburgers and fries were always a constant temptation.

Waiting for Spring

I shiver as the wind blows signal digits up my sleeves.
This interminable winter is a greedy guest
who has forgotten to go home.

Hat down to my eyebrows, jacket zipped to my chin,
scarf snug in place, I walk the frozen roadside,
wishing my parents were young again,
wishing they didn't need my care.
Yet somehow, I will still find joy.

The clouds above are cynical sentinels,
but I choose to smile anyway.
God watches over us,
and spring has already bought her ticket home.

I Corinthians 13:7

"Love never gives up; and its faith, hope, and patience never fail."

The Difference a Day Makes

I had been worried about Mom's lungs, but the chest x-ray came back normal. In fact her doctor called me early in the morning with the news that my mother was awake and trying to talk. He felt the next day he would send her home from the hospital. I was surprised to hear she was doing so much better, and also I was depressed.

It was easy for me to figure out why I suddenly felt depressed. My mother would be home the next day. This meant the long, hard work of keeping Mom safe and well was continuing. Bill and I were still trapped by responsibility, now more than ever since Mom had become so frail. We could not move near our children yet; and we could not visit our grandson anytime soon. With Mom's physical condition the way it was, Bill and I decided we would not want to leave her alone with our assistant. There was just too much for one person to worry about.

Even our assistant would have more responsibilities now that Mom needed extra care. Since I couldn't pay her for the added work of changing Mom's bandages and overseeing the catheter, I told her she could leave an hour earlier each evening. I knew the extra hour at home was something she would enjoy, but this meant that Bill and I would need to feed my mother supper every night. Now we would have even less freedom.

In one of Joyce Meyer's books, she suggests that if you don't understand why a hardship takes so long to go away, it is wise to look for what God is trying to teach you. This made me think of the great lesson on love written by Paul to the Corinthians. He writes that love is patient.

According to the definition of patience in the dictionary, I was not patient. Too often I complained to Bill and my closest friends. Too often I found myself restless and unhappy. I was not at peace with the job that God had guided me to do.

Patience also means steadfastness. To me this meant I should not allow my thoughts to shilly-shally back and forth between wanting and not wanting to do this job. I knew I'd be more peaceful if I willingly accepted my job as caregiver.

Just writing these thoughts out in my journal helped me to focus my thoughts in a more positive direction. My spirit felt much lighter. Also I continued to tell myself, *All is as it should be. God is in charge.* I believed God would decide the right time to change things. He loved each one of us and knew what was best for us now and in the future.

Certainly I needed to continue my study of I Corinthians 13. After all, the most important attribute was love for God and others. If I could understand how to be at peace while I loved my mother by being her caregiver, I'd be less upset and depressed.

YOUR JOURNAL

Read I Corinthian 13. What part comes naturally to you? Which one needs the most work?

TIP FOR CAREGIVER

When my parents moved in with Bill and me, they decided it would be a good idea to meet with a lawyer at the Office of the Aging. His services were completely free for seniors. At the time, they signed revised wills, living wills, and appointed me Power of Attorney and Health Care Proxy.

A good thing Power of Attorney was in place because it wasn't long before I had to pay my parents' bills, cash their checks, and do their banking. This document made it easier for me as I took on their financial responsibilities.

Learned Response

When I wanted Mom and Dad's attention,
I got it.
When my mate and I wanted children,
we had them.
When we wanted a house,
we bought one.

I am tired of being a caregiver,
but the job continues anyway.
No wonder I feel like something is wrong.

Psalm 139:5-6

"You are all around me on every side;
   you protect me with your power.
Your knowledge of me is too deep;
   it is beyond my understanding."

Another Infection

This morning my mother was supposed to come home from the hospital, but something was wrong. Our assistant and I discovered the urine in her catheter tube was milky. We have learned from past experience that when my mother's urine becomes cloudy, this is a sure sign of a urinary tract infection. We brought this problem to the attention of the nurse who then called the doctor. A urine sample would be taken and tested.

My mother was so sleepy that we could not feed her or give her liquids. How could we possibly take her home in this condition? It was frustrating to know that she had an infection, but could not be treated until proven by lab results. My recent inspirational reading and prayer helped me to remember that God is trustworthy; and He would guide the doctor in my mother's best interest.

If she came home, we would do the best we could. Perhaps we would have to give her liquids through an eyedropper if this was necessary to keep her hydrated. When the results of the urine culture came back positive, the doctor would order the appropriate medication, and hopefully, Mom would start to get better again.

About 9 AM our caregiver called from the hospital. My mother would not come home this day. She did not have enough sodium in her blood so she would need intravenous treatment to correct this problem.

Now I felt more relaxed. The next day preliminary results of the culture would come back from the lab. Then if she were released from the hospital, she would come home with oral medication. In the meantime if the urinary tract infection gave her a high temperature, most likely the doctor would begin an antibiotic immediately anyway.

There was a benefit to this new development; she would be on the super expensive, hi-tech alternating air mattress another day. Since she had been on this mattress, her wounds appeared to have improved, yet once she was home on an inferior alternating air mattress, I did not know if she would continue to heal.

With all the problems we had recently with the thin mattress hospice had provided, Bill decided to order our own much better alternating air mattress. The order was placed on the Internet, and the company would ship it to our house. Later, Bill would try to get a reimbursement from Medicare.

I continued to trust God. He would continue to orchestrate every aspect my mother's care. He alone knew what was best for her.

YOUR JOURNAL

When you are disappointed about something, what do you tell yourself?

TIP FOR CAREGIVER

I discovered that when my mother was in the hospital, her assistant and I needed to be extremely alert to changes in her condition. When she had a catheter, we had to watch the urine in the tube and bag to make sure it didn't change in color, a sign of an infection. Doctors and nurses are busy and in a hurry so sometimes they overlook something important.

Bewildered

When I gazed at our dark maple tree,
I did not know he would cut it down.
Now there is a stump in place of its beauty.

When Mom got another bad infection,
I did not know she would die.
Now there is an empty hole in my heart.

Psalm 145:17-20a

"The LORD is righteous in all he does,
    merciful in all his acts.
He is near to those who call to him,
    who call to him with sincerity.
He supplies the needs of those who honor him;
    he hears their cries and saves them.
He protects everyone who loves him . . ."

Two Days Later

The doctor ordered my mother another chest x-ray because he felt she was a bit congested. Also our assistant found out that nurses had been giving Mom cough medication. There was a good chance that the reason Mom had been so sleepy at times and difficult to feed was due to this medication. Also the doctor ordered another swallowing test.

Now I was angry. The first week Mom was in the hospital, I told her doctor that I did not want her to have another swallowing test. Not too long ago, she had had this test. It determined she needed a special diet and thick liquids. Our assistant and I had discovered though that once Mom felt better and got stronger, there did not seem to be a need to keep her on this diet. If the cough medication was causing her to be sleepy, then the solution was not another swallowing test.

After I spoke with the doctor voicing my concerns, he cancelled the cough medicine and the test. This made me think of all the poor people that are very sick or very old that do not have an advocate by their side. They end up with medication and tests that may be unnecessary. They end up with feeding tubes that aren't always in their best interest. What an education Bill, our assistant, and I had acquired by caring for my parents.

*

On this same day, as I drove into the hospital parking garage, I asked God to find me a good space. The day before there had been extremely slim pickings. Today I was agitated and angry with all that was going on with my mother, so I felt I needed a little extra help.

As I drove up to the roof, there were no spaces along the way, but I held the thought that there would be a good space for me right near the door. Lo and behold, just as I had thought, it was there, waiting for me. I praised God! I knew He wanted me to know He was there and continued to watch over me. God's blessings were all around me; I only had to see them for what they were.

YOUR JOURNAL

What has God done for you and your loved one recently that you praised and thanked Him for?

TIP FOR CAREGIVER

Shortly after my mother entered the hospital, I took her off hospice. This meant that Medicare would now cover all those tests and hi-tech procedures she had in an attempt to save her life. However, months later my husband had to make many telephone calls to untangle the misconception by Medicare that my mother was still on hospice during her hospital stay. I am glad my husband had the time and patience to accomplish this feat.

Unseen Truth

Today it is cloudy, but
the sun is still there.
Winter trees are bare, but
soon they will be full and green.
I don't see my Savior's face, but
I know that He is with me.

Psalm 18:4-6

"The danger of death was all around me;
   the waves of destruction rolled over me.
The danger of death was around me,
   and the grave set its trap for me.
In my trouble I called to the Lord;
   I called to my God for help.
In his temple he heard my voice;
   he listened to my cry for help."

Not out of Options

Once again our assistant told me that my mother was sleepy, and it was hard to get any food or liquids into her. Since my mother's urine collection bag was low, our assistant worried that my mother would suffer from dehydration.

Later when I spoke to the doctor on the telephone, he said that he wanted to send her home, but he would wait for the results of yet another chest x-ray. I explained how hard it was to feed her and give her liquids. *She'll die if you send her home now*, I told him. He asked me if I might want to put her into a nursing home, and my answer was she could get better care at home.

Shortly after I spoke with the doctor, a nurse called me to say my mother would definitely be coming home. Immediately I called the case manager who told me that if my mother needed to leave the hospital with an intravenous drip to treat her UTI and provide hydration, she would have to go to a nursing home. Medicare would not pay for a nurse to come to the house every day to monitor the intravenous medication. I told her that my mother was not eating or drinking. The case manager said that she would speak to the doctor.

Two positive things did happen right away. Finally my mother was put on a long overdue antibiotic for her UTI. Hopefully, now she would become more alert. Also, the case manager told our assistant who was still at Mom's bedside that we were not out of options yet. This new development with the UTI would allow Medicare to keep paying for my mother's stay in the hospital. *What a relief!*

After I got into the car to leave for the hospital, I felt too upset to drive there. I went back in the house and decided to stay home. I decided I needed break from the hospital. There had been too many ups and downs and not such good surprises around every curve lately. The journey had been hard as I watched my mother come near death and then get better only to see her decline once again. Still I would trust God because He knew what was best for Mom.

YOUR JOURNAL

Have you ever felt tired and discouraged to the point of needing to ask for someone's help in doing your job?

TIP FOR CAREGIVER

I discovered that visiting my mother in the hospital could be extremely tiring and draining emotionally and physically. This was the time I needed to listen to my instincts. If I needed to stay home and rest, I did. If I needed to ask our assistant to go to the hospital instead of me, I did. If Bill and I needed to eat out, bring in take-out food, or open up a can of soup, we did. I was just barely getting through the trauma of watching my mother's health go up and down without adding housecleaning and cooking to the mix.

Both Sides

Spring is here, but
the yard is still brown and barren.
The birds have returned, but
the warmer temperatures
are stalled somewhere on I-95.

One minute there is hope, but
the next my mother is near death
One minute I'm a caregiver, but
the next I'm not sure who I will be.

Proverbs 9:8-9

"Never correct conceited people; they will hate you for it. But if you correct the wise, they will respect you. Anything you say to the wise will make them wiser. Whatever you tell the righteous will add to their knowledge."

The Guidance I Needed

God's guidance came even when I did not know I needed it. My mother had been in the hospital for about three weeks. I had become completely frustrated by some of her doctor's decisions, and every time I had to call him I dreaded it. He seemed impatient with my questions or suggestions. At one point, a nurse called him with one of my questions, and he hung up on her. My assistant and I had observed things that he seemed to miss when he examined her such as an allergic reaction to an antibiotic, the cloudiness of her urine, and the swelling of her arm. When I was there, he stood in the room and talked with me briefly without coming near my mother.

In my opinion, he relied too heavily on the nurses' observations. Of course, the nurses were extremely busy which meant sometimes important changes were not caught until our assistant and I came to visit. Mom's doctor never explained why he had wanted to send her home when she couldn't eat or drink and still had a urinary tract infection. His decision had seemed illogical to Bill, our assistant, and I. If he felt there was nothing more he could do for her, I would have thought he should discuss this with me. Perhaps he did not want to make the time to sit with me a few minutes and discuss her condition.

God knew how confused and frustrated I had become, and He sent me the help I needed. An "angel" who worked at the hospital told me that recently her mother had passed away. Her own experience had given her true compassion as she listened to my complaints about my mother's doctor. Then she gave me the information that I desperately needed. Even though this was something she was *not allowed to do*, she suggested we might want to turn my mother's case over to the hospital doctors. She said that these doctors work as a team 24 hours a day and 7 days a week, and they would not leave any stone unturned.

Bill and I made the decision to let go of Mom's doctor and let this team of doctors take over. My mother's nurse oversaw the transition, not allowing it to take any longer than necessary. That same day a young doctor came to speak with me. She had already reviewed my mother's records and had a clear grasp of what had transpired during my mother's long stay at the hospital. For at least fifteen to twenty minutes, we discussed my mother's condition and the options available.

My confidence level in the mother's care went from zero to as high as it could go. First my mother was given some added medication intravenously, vitamins and a blood thinner which she could no longer take orally and a second medication for her UTI. Her new doctor had explained to me that my mother not only had a bacterial infection but also a fungal infection.

Later a neurologist was also called in to evaluate Mom's dementia. He would try to determine how much of a part this dementia played in her continued listlessness and disinterest in food and liquids.

Again the swallowing test was suggested, and this time I did allow it. The results were extremely poor. My mother had reached a point of no ability to swallow anything. This was extremely upsetting to me. However I did feel good about one thing. I felt that I had made the right decision to ask new doctors to take over her case. I sensed they would do everything possible.

I still understood that given my mother's age and the severity of her recent infections, no matter what was being done for her might not be enough, but at least she now had a chance. It was easy for me to sense God's guidance. At just the right moment, a good person had come along with the information I needed. *Thank you, dear God.*

YOUR JOURNAL

If someone seemed to magically appear before you with just the right information at just the right time, what would you think?

TIP FOR CAREGIVER

Our assistant and I always took the attitude that doctors had their medical training, but we were the ones who knew George and Mom best. We would respectfully voice our opinion if the doctor said or ordered something that we did not understand or did not agree with. We understood that doctors are busy, and like everyone else they can make mistakes. Sometimes they are unable to make a wise decision unless someone close to the patient is willing to offer what they know. The best doctors are the ones who don't think they are always right and are willing to listen to a caregiver's point of view, even if the caregiver does not have a medical degree.

No Rest

The road is now straight up,
no gentle slopes downward for rest,
and yet I try to do my best.
Maybe I no longer care.
Maybe my love's worn bare.
Dear Lord, please hear my earnest prayer.

Psalm 139:15-16

"When my bones were being formed,
   carefully put together in my mother's womb,
when I was growing there in secret,
   you knew that I was there—
   you saw me before I was born.
The days allotted to me
   had all been recorded in your book,
   before any of them ever began."

Holding On and Letting Go

At the beginning of my mother's four-week hospital stay, I thought eventually she would return to the way she was before her illness. Then the pendulum swung, and she became so weak I thought she would die. Then the pendulum swung ever so slightly, and she improved enough to consume minute amounts of thickened liquids and pureed foods. However soon it became obvious she could not consume enough nourishment to stay alive.

According to her doctor, Mom's swallowing reflex was almost non-existent, and the risk of aspirating her food into her lungs was high. This meant she could easily develop pneumonia. Since I did not want to put her on a feeding tube, there was no other alternative but continue to spoon-feed her as best as possible.

Now I understood why families put their elderly parents on feeding tubes. No one wants to see his or her parent slowly starve to death, including me. I personally felt though that my mother's dementia had reached such an advanced stage that keeping her alive artificially might not be in her best interest. She was extremely prone to infection and her sores could worsen, becoming infected again. A peaceful, pain free death was what I was hoped for, unless she rallied to the point that she could eat healthy portions of food again.

I had no idea how my mother would be from day to day and whether she would ever come home again. This not knowing, along with a growing sense of helplessness, made me anxious and restless. It was difficult to concentrate on anything else.

When I reminded myself God was in charge, I felt much better. No matter what I did or did not do, no matter what the doctor's tried or did not try, it was a comfort to know that my mother was safe in God's care. He would decide what would happen to her and whether it was her time to be with Him in heaven. Another thought that I found helpful was once Mom was in heaven her spirit would be free from dementia, and she would return back to normal. She'd be herself again. Now this was good news.

YOUR JOURNAL

When was the last time you sensed God's wisdom, guidance, or protection in the life of your loved one?

TIP FOR CAREGIVER

When I was losing my peace, prayer and talking to my most positive girlfriend often did wonders. The worst thing I could do was to sing the blues, *Poor me. Poor me.* Feeling sorry for myself was never, ever a good thing. It only made me feel worse.

The Monster

Just when you're about to sleep,
the Monster comes with corkscrew teeth.
He bores deep inside your brain,
making you go quite insane.

It forces you to ask, *Did I dot every i;*
is the truth a bold face lie?
The more you think about it,
the more you want to die.

Then above its sickening sound,
you hear a clear, kind voice,
With God all things are possible, but
it's still your choice.

You decide to ask for help,
trust God with all your might,
remembering our Heavenly Father
sends peace both day or night.

The Monster twists much faster
than it did before, but
this time it breaks free and
flees towards the door.

Now when you close your eyes,
there is nothing to fear.
When the monster arrives,
you will fight with prayer.

Romans 8:26-27

"... the Spirit also comes to help us, weak as we are. For we do not know how we ought to pray; the Spirit himself pleads with God for us in groans that words cannot express. And God, who sees into our hearts, knows what the thought of the Spirit is; because the Spirit pleads with God on behalf of his people and in accordance with his will."

Good Can Come From Bad

My mother continued to be weak and unable to drink and eat food even after a full regime of antibiotics for her UTI. According to one of new doctors and the case manager, my mother's dementia had taken a large dip downward, and she was not expected to rally. Time was running out for me to keep her in the hospital because her antibiotic treatment was almost through. Medicare would not continue to pay for her to be there, and if I took her home on an intravenous drip to continue to hydrate her, Medicare would not pay for a nurse to come in and monitor the IV on a daily basis.

We did consider hiring someone out of my mother's money in her bank account, but the doctor and case manager basically talked me out of it. My mother was very weak, and there was a real possibility she would continue to develop infections in her wounds or come down with pneumonia. Her swallowing reflex was almost non-existent. They recommend that I take her off the IV and when necessary put her on morphine to keep her comfortable.

I was told that if I didn't put my mother back on hospice, I would have to take her out of the hospital right away. With hospice coming, there was a possibility I could keep her there longer. This appealed to me because I felt at the hospital Mom would continue to be kept comfortable, and I would be less worried and stressed.

Again I thought about why many elderly people with severe dementia end up in with a feeding tube. For some daughters and sons the decision to slowly watch their parent die is never an option. Probably there are many other reasons why a feeding tube is chosen as the way to go. Now I knew first hand that this is a caregiver's hardest decision. It certainly was mine.

I asked an internist on my mother's case what he thought I should do. His said the kindest thing to do was to take her off the IV and let her die. He said given the same circumstance this is the decision he would make for someone in his own family.

After the doctor was gone, questions remained in my mind about whether we had tried everything. Next time I saw him, I would discuss this issue, but I suspected there would always be a lingering doubt in my mind and heart no matter what he said. It is human nature to feel that something might be missed when it comes down to matters of life and death.

I asked my friends to pray that my mother would not suffer and for God's continued guidance and wisdom for Bill, our assistant, and myself. My prayer had been that God would take my mother *clean and fast*, but for some reason He had said no. It would not be clean because the decision whether to use a feeding tube was muddy, complicated, filled with guilt and doubt. It would not be fast because she would slowly dehydrate to death.

It occurred to me that God in his wisdom had a good reason why things didn't turn out as I had hoped they would. There was a positive in this horrible, horrible walk through my mother's end-stage dementia. God, Mom, and I would forever be partners, helping others to understand their own feelings, thoughts, and prayers as they went through similar circumstances. Perhaps my writings would help someone remember: *You are not alone. Others tread these waters. God is with you; He will guide you to make the right decision for your loved one and send you His peace.*

YOUR JOURNAL

Who will help you today with your loved one so you can get some free time. Remember, no one can succeed as a caregiver without lots of help.

TIP FOR CAREGIVER

When George's legs became weak, he still wanted to use his walker instead of a wheelchair when he got up to go to the bathroom. I tried to keep his wheelchair nearby in case he needed to sit down in a hurry. It was in a locked position, so it wouldn't slide away from him.

The Three of Us

Side-by-side we walk for miles,
sometimes climbing mountains,
other times pushing
through thorny bushes.
We reach the darkest woods
where there is a fork in the road.
You take the road to heaven,
and I take the other, but
you and I are not alone.

James 3:17

" . . . the wisdom from above is pure first of all; it is also peaceful, gentle, and friendly; it is full of compassion and produces a harvest of good deeds; it is free from prejudice and hypocrisy."

Letting Go

It finally started: the process of letting my mother go. All intravenous support was stopped. My thoughts and emotions were a tangled mess. In my mind, the intravenous was Mom's last vestige of hope, but without a feeding tube to keep her alive, there was no need for the IV. This was done because the IV drip would only cause more problems since my mother's dying body soon would not be able to handle the liquid any more. Even though I understood this, it didn't make it any easier to see my symbol of hope taken away.

Then I reminded myself that my mother was ninety-years-old. She was weak, and she would keep getting infections or worsening bedsores. I was being kind by letting her go. Her inability to swallow was a sign that her life was coming to an end. I read in a booklet that my pastor gave me that other cultures don't even think of a feeding tube for their elderly. For some reason I found this comforting.

The lady from hospice came so I could sign my mother back into the program. She told me that my mother could stay in the hospital until hospice felt ready to support her at home.

In her weakened state, I thought my mother would immediately run a temperature and show signs of dehydration. My prayer was that she would die quickly, and I would not have to take her home. This was my wish for her sake as well as mine. Also I prayed that she would die without discomfort. I knew this could be done with the help of morphine.

I reminded myself that God was ultimately in charge. If He wanted her to live, she would still be able to swallow, and the doctors would not have said there was no hope of her returning to good health.

Of course, there was still doubt in my mind. It was hard to rid myself of the thought that if Mom were put on a feeding tube she would become strong and able to swallow again. The doctors cautioned me though that even if she did get stronger, bedsores and infection would continue to be a problem, and she would suffer.

I had counted on the antibiotics and the IV to make her better. Then I had counted on the sheer determination of Bill, our assistant, and I get her to swallow fluids and food. But now I had to admit nothing had worked the way I thought it might, yet I was still reluctant to give up. I wished we could give her another chance by keeping her on intravenous another week, but we had come to the end of the line. Medicare refused to pay for her hospital stay any longer because the doctors felt that there was nothing more they could do for her. This time she would not rally and get better. End-stage dementia had brought her to the point of not being able to swallow, and this meant she would die.

*

The last day my mother was in the hospital, two of her doctors spoke to me again. I believe God made sure I was at the right place, at the right time, to meet with them at my mother's bedside. First the neurologist explained that even if my mother did rally and regain her swallowing, she would soon become ill because her body was failing. He felt that by not inserting a feeding tube, I was doing the kindest thing I could do for her.

The internist who had been following my mother's case for about four days came in next. He explained that even if we missed something that this was only ten percent of the picture. The eighty percent left would not change the fact that my mother couldn't swallow and her body was failing. He also felt I was making the right decision.

I had faith that God was still orchestrating everything regarding my mother's care. I had prayed that I would speak when necessary, and I had spoken. God had guided me and would continue to guide me.

YOUR JOURNAL

How do you feel about your care giving commitment today?

TIP FOR CAREGIVER

After I prayed for God's guidance and after I asked the opinion of my mother's doctors, I should have had complete peace about my decision against a feeding tube, but I didn't. I had a hard time with it and still do.

I urge you, the caregiver, to think about end-of-life decisions you might have to make. If your loved one has a living will and you are the health proxy, all you need to do is follow his or her wishes found in the legal document, right? But what if this legal document doesn't cover what is best for your loved one? What decision will you make then?

If there is no living will, my personal recommendation would be to start thinking about how you feel about extending life with medical equipment such respirators and feeding tubes when the prognosis for quality of life is not good. Many caregivers have no problem saying no to medical intervention when they know their loved one would only continue to become ill and suffer in the near future.

Truthfully, if I could have a do over, I would probably make a different decision. Since my mother didn't seem to be suffering or in pain, I would let her have the feeding tube. Even though the doctor's said she would not have a good quality of life, I'd give her this one last chance. *Hindsight!* It seems so easy to make a different decision after the fact, but whether it would have been a kinder, better decision is still debatable.

I realize the above somewhat contradicts what I have written on this subject, but all I can say, is this is where I am as I finish writing this book. This does not mean I have finally discovered the truth. It only means this is where my journey has taken me so far.

Waiting

I prayed for quick and clean,
but God knows what is best.
Her death seems much too slow,
but He knows the right time.

Psalm 23: 1-4

"The Lord is my shepherd;
   I have everything I need.
He lets me rest in fields of green grass
   and leads me to quiet pools of fresh water.
He gives me new strength.
He guides me in the right paths,
   as he has promised.
Even if I go through the deepest darkness,
   I will not be afraid, Lord,
     for you are with me.
Your shepherd's rod and staff protect me."

The Wait

    Mom's IV had been stopped on a Wednesday afternoon while she was still in the hospital. It had been the worse day of my life. Now there was no hope for her to live. The doctor had told me she would dehydrate, and it would take about a week for her to die.

    Hospice could no long keep my mother in the hospital because Medicare would no longer pay for her to be there. I became afraid of what was ahead. Surely the next few days would be extremely difficult as I took charge of her care again only to watch her die.

    My mother's doctor gave hospice a prescription for liquid Morphine that was delivered to the house the same day my mother came home. It was to be administered under her tongue as needed.

    A hospice nurse and social worker came the very next day. Of course there was little the nurse could do at this point, but it was comfort for me to know she would be available any time my assistant or I had questions and concerns.

    It was also a comfort seeing my mother covered with her own sheets and blankets in her own bed, but soon enough I realized nothing could prepare me for how hard it would be to watch her die.

    At first our assistant and I offered her minute amounts of baby food fruit and thickened liquids, being careful that she did not choke. It soon became apparent to us that she could not swallow anything.

The best we could do was just wet her mouth with swabs, and even then we had to be very careful that drops didn't roll down her throat and choke her. I didn't want her to die that way.

Bill visited my mother often throughout the day, but either our assistant or I stayed near her bed all the time. At night after our assistant went home, Bill and I kept the monitor in our bedroom on the highest volume. We both woke up often, listening to the pattern of my mother's breathing. I was afraid I'd miss a change that would signal she was near death. I wanted to be able to administer morphine if she began to struggle for air. From experience with my stepfather, I knew this drug would relax her breathing muscles, making it easier for her to breath.

I soon realized that it was good my mother was home rather than in the hospital. I spent lots of time with her and had the comfort of my own food, shower, and bed.

The last twenty-four hours of Mom's life, our assistant and I stayed with her around the clock. We began administering a small amount of morphine under her tongue when she appeared restless. We had been told that her body would instantly absorb the morphine, but this did not happen. This very small amount of liquid was running to the back of her throat and caused her to start choking. We couldn't understand why.

We called the hospice nurse on duty for the evening, and it was determined that the wrong type of morphine had been delivered to our house. The one we had was a weaker dose for those patients who could still swallow. Immediately the right medication was ordered, and the hospice nurse came out in horrible weather to deliver it to us. *God bless her.*

After we had the right medication, we were able to administer it to my mother every two hours without any problems. The morphine relaxed her, making her breathing easier. In fact, when the nurse and social worker from hospice came on Monday morning, they both told me that my mother was not suffering. They said there was no stress in the expression on her face, and she was peaceful. *She's in a good place*, the nurse said. I'll never forget those words. *She's in a good place.*

After the nurse left, our assistant and I both felt that my mother would die soon. It was now the sixth day since my mother had been taken off intravenous fluids, and extreme dehydration was evident. Her breathing had become more strained and there were longer pauses between breaths.

As we sat in my mother's room, our assistant and I found ourselves acting silly and joking around. What was wrong with us that we could do this with a dying woman who we loved right there?

Shortly after I observed our strange behavior, Pastor Gloria called. I updated her on my mother's condition, and then I found myself asking her how our assistant and I could be so silly at such a sad time. Immediately she made me feel better by saying it was a human trait, a way of releasing tension. I was relieved that we hadn't lost our minds.

Later that day my mother took her last breaths. She was gone. I hugged her as she lay there. I said my goodbyes, so did Bill and our assistant. I wanted to cry, but I didn't, a weird side-effect of the antidepressant that I was on. It would have been better if I could have cried.

Bill, our assistant, Pastor Gloria, and I sat down at the table to have a bite to eat, but I was not at ease. I wondered if I was acting strangely again. How could I eat and talk normally while, a few steps away, was my mother's body? I also felt ill at ease, waiting for the undertaker to pick her up. Everything felt like a surreal experience.

At some point, I felt compelled to see my mother one last time in her own bed. I kissed her now cooling body and her pale face, and I said goodbye again. I'm not sure that was good for me because later it did add one more sad memory.

YOUR JOURNAL

What is your most earnest and reoccurring prayer for your loved one? Why?

TIP FOR CAREGIVER

There is no right or wrong way to feel or act when our loved one dies. Just so long as we don't hurt the living or ourselves, we are free to respond in a multitude of ways. These are all acceptable: shock, numbness, intense pain, delayed pain, laughter, tears, happiness, sadness, hunger, no-appetite, hyperactivity, laziness, sleep, insomnia, etc. There is no perfect way to watch those we love die and no set way to mourn them after they are gone.

Spring Won't Wait

The bees buzz among cherry blossoms,
and a purple finch nests on an electric lantern

under our deck. These mix with memories
of my mother's last breaths.

Spring won't wait for me to fall asleep easily
or awake without feeling something is wrong.

The sun's rays have already shifted, and God will
continue to reveal His plan for each day

while Magnolia petals open, then drop
one by one on the grass.

I Peter 5:8-11

"Be alert, be on watch! Your enemy, the Devil, roams around like a roaring lion, looking for someone to devour. Be firm in your faith and resist him, because you know that the other believers in all the world are going through the same kind of sufferings. But after you have suffered for a little while, the God of all grace, who calls you to share his eternal glory in union with Christ, will himself perfect you and give you firmness, strength, and a sure foundation. To him be the power forever! Amen."

In Search of Peace

Now that my stepfather and my mother were in heaven, the job God had given me was over. I no longer carried the huge weight of responsibility that I carried all these years. Without Bill and our assistant, I would have never been able to finish this work. All praise goes to God for protecting my parents and guiding the three of us as we took care of them.

Now it was time to mourn my mother's passing. A month after she died, I missed her intensely, but I did not miss all the work and worry of taking care of her. I missed seeing her, holding her hand, and talking to her. I missed the occasional words she would say. I missed her smile, the lift of her eyebrows, the nod of her head, the shrug of her shoulders. All those little movements that showed me she was still there, still communicating with me. Even though dementia had taken most of her away from me, I missed the good feeling I had when I was with her. Somehow we had communicated our love for each other, especially when I kissed and hugged her. We were still mother and daughter to the end.

Even though I listened to the doctors' recommendation not to give my mother a feeding tube, I still had what I called "irrational guilt" about it. I also had some real guilt mixed in there as well, so I decided to write about my thoughts, hoping I could analyze them dispassionately. Maybe then I would understand my decision and not feel guilty anymore.

*

My mother could not swallow food or liquids anymore. This is a condition that is found in people with end-stage dementia. It often occurs after an infection. My mother had two infections back to back, and she could no longer take in any nourishment. Without the feeding tube she would die.

Two of my mother's doctors recommended against the feeding tube. They said she would continue to get infections in her wounds, and the feeding tube could actually cause infection and aspiration of her lungs. Her quality of life would not be good, and she would suffer. One doctor said that it would kinder for my mother if I did not choose a feeding tube.

At the same time I made this decision against the feeding tube for my mother, I was tired of taking care of her, and I wished the job were over. I wanted freedom from this huge responsibility. There was a part of me that was relieved that this commitment was ending.

Even though I understood my mother's inability to swallow was what caused her death, I still felt I gave her a death sentence sooner rather than later. All these years, she counted on me to protect her as if she were my little child. How could I decide against a feeding tube and just stand back and let her die?

As I write the above, my sense of guilt comes from my negative feelings at the time I was making this difficult decision. If my intense desire for freedom wasn't there, would I have made the same decision? This is the torture of looking back.

Of course I can always speculate. I think I would have made the same decision of no feeding tube because both doctors on my mother's case agreed that I had to let her go in order to prevent more suffering. And yes, I know if my decision was done without any of my own selfish feelings getting in the way, it would have definitely been easier.

It is becoming clear to me that I must stop analyzing all of this. I must leave all this second-guessing and all these painful doubts with God. He will forgive all my wrong motives and thoughts. Anything that was not done purely out of love for my mother is forgiven. And ultimately it was God's decision that He took her to heaven. I do not have the power of life and death; only God has this power.

My dear husband and others have reminded me that I went above and beyond the call of duty, taking care of both my parents at home. They have told me that I should feel good about what I did for them all these years. They say that I made the very best decision I could for my mother regarding a feeding tube.

I just pray that God will help me to forgive myself for some very human thoughts and emotions that were there at the same time I needed to make a wise decision for my mother.

I know Satan wants to destroy my peace, but God wants me to have deep peace. God wants me to feel good about what I did right all these nine years for my parents and not concentrate on this one last decision.

YOUR JOURNAL

Have you ever felt intensely guilty for something you said or did? Do you think your guilt was justified or irrational?

TIP FOR CAREGIVER

After my mother passed away, I was relieved that I did not have to do unpleasant caregiver duties ever again. Now Bill and I could visit our children and grandchild whenever we wanted. Instead of feeling guilty about this, I knew it was a normal, human thing to celebrate our freedom from the heavy responsibility that had lasted so long. Other the other hand, I missed my mother intensely because I loved her and always will. I'm glad that I was able to allow feelings of both joy and sadness to co-exist in peace.

Your Picture

I stand in your kitchen
and suffocate with grief.
For fifty-nine years you gave me
unconditional love,
but now this place is empty.

Back on my side of the house,
your picture on the refrigerator
reminds me in this life
there is loss and pain.

No longer do I spoon-feed you,
wash you top to bottom, and
worry over your chronic wounds.
Finally freedom has come
at too high a cost.

John 3:16-17

"For God loved the world so much that he gave his only Son, so that everyone who believes in him may not die but have eternal life. For God did not send his Son into the world to be its judge, but to be its savior."

God's Grace

God knew how hard it has been for me to live with my decision about the feeding tube. I believe this is why He made sure I heard about two examples of elderly folks who were put on feeding tubes unsuccessfully. One case was an elderly man in a nursing home who received a feeding tube only to die shortly after. Another case was an elderly woman who had been my mother's roommate at the hospital. She was put on a feeding tube but began to have serious medical problems with it. Later the feeding tube was taken out, and her family had to let her go.

*

It was the early part of September. My mother had died in April. The pain of losing her was still deep and raw. I had a hard time going over to my parent's side of the house where they lived out the last nine years of their life. Their presence seemed so strong there that I was reminded of my loss and how very much I missed them. Also I was reminded of how frail and helpless they had become over the years.

A few months after my mother's death, I talked to my pastor about my reoccurring feelings of guilt regarding my decision against the feeding tube.

What do I tell myself?" I asked her.

You are forgiven, she said simply.

Perhaps I did nothing wrong and everything right for my mother, but if my selfish desire for my freedom somehow tainted my decision, I was still forgiven. Our Lord Jesus died on the cross as a sacrifice for my sins. What a wonderful comfort. What a complete peace.

*

Now Bill and I were free to go on a long vacation, something we hadn't done in a long time. We bought a travel trailer and a commercial van to pull it and off we went for a camping trip in Alabama. It was the month of March, and we were looking forward to spring temperatures that come early in this part of the country.

Surrounded by tall, long-leafed pines at the campground, God spoke to me in my heart and mind. He told me that I could not understand *now* why I denied my mother a feeding tube because I was a different person *back then*. I took this to mean that my mother's severe decline, the doctor's suggestions, and my state of mind had all gone into who I was then and why I made this decision. Now that this horrible circumstance was in the past, I had changed and could no longer understand the person I was back then and why I made the decision against a feeding tube. Now I should be kind to myself and not torture myself with a question that I no longer had the ability to answer. I found great comfort in this thought.

Praise God! He sends His peace. He still takes care of me.

YOUR JOURNAL

What does it mean to you that Jesus our Lord and Savior died on a cross for your sins so you may be forgiven?

TIP FOR CAREGIVER

After both my parents passed away, Bill and I were still using their refrigerator for overflow items. It made me sad to walk through their part of the house. Each time I felt like my heart was about to break until I devised a way I could overcome the horrible grief. I spoke to myself as I made my way to the refrigerator. *They are in heaven. They are now strong, well, and happy.* This chant of sorts made it almost bearable to be surrounded by so many intense memories.

Ducks at Eufaula National Wildlife Refuge

We hike, taking in the smell of pine
and unfamiliar bird calls.
At Lookout Tower a beehive hums loudly.
We leave in a hurry, but not before observing
black ducks in the flooded field below.

Later I flip through the field guide but
can't find those ducks.
It is frustrating, just like memories
that can't absolve me from denying
my mother a feeding tube.
Back then her doctors said, *This is a kind thing
to do, so she won't suffer,* but why didn't I
give her one more chance?
How could I just let her die?

The other day God gave me a revelation;
that I shouldn't torture myself
since circumstances back then
made me a different person.
The page with a clear explanation
is no longer available . . .

nor will I find the right species
in the field guide. The name
black ducks will have to do.

Psalm 100:5

"The Lord is good;
 his love is eternal
 and his faithfulness lasts forever."

Last Thoughts

If I were magically transported back nine years with all my memories intact, would I take care of my parents at home again? My immediate answer is *No way!* It was a hard, long road that became even more difficult toward the end. Back then, however, I came to believe that God wanted me to do this job. He sent me all the help and encouragement that I needed along the way, yet right now *only His power* could convince me to do it all over again.

Now I understand why people must put their loved ones in nursing homes. If a daughter or a son doesn't have the space in their house, doesn't have the money to hire outside help, doesn't have a spouse that is willing to help, or doesn't have the stomach for it, there is nothing left to do but to look for a good nursing home. Hopefully, there are good ones out there.

I continue to believe that God took me on this nine-year journey, so I could grow into a more compassionate and caring person. Now I realize that life can be almost impossible for many people, both young and old. This means we all need a helping hand especially when things get tough.

Even with all the help God provided me, I still found myself praying for a better attitude. By turning to God often and by looking to Him for answers in inspirational books, sermons, and the promptings of the Holy Spirit, I became closer to Him. I felt His presence. He was teaching me to rely on Him for guidance and enthusiasm each day.

God was also teaching me to be more like His Son, Jesus, who loved perfectly. Although my transformation will never be complete in this life, caring for my parents with the help of the Holy Spirit, I learned lessons on how to love God and others.

Surely, God guided me to write this book even though at first it was the last thing I wanted to do. It seemed much too depressing to write about my life as a caregiver. At first, I was only able to express myself in poems, and then slowly but surely I began writing prose too. God knew how to bring me along to do His will by sharing my experiences.

Hopefully this book has helped you in some small way to understand what it is like to take care of a loved one at home, how hard and exhausting it can be at times, what some of your feelings and thoughts might be along the way, and how one other person was able to make it through.

If this book does nothing else, at the very least I hope it has made you feel you are not alone. I have been there. Others have been there. And if you ask Him, God will be with you every step of the way. He will tread water with you, keeping your head above the water, as you take care of your parents at home.

YOUR JOURNAL

Are you still convinced God wants you to be a caregiver to your loved one or do you think God is guiding you to make other plans?

TIP FOR CAREGIVER

Always remember, God takes care of us and sends his wisdom and help in many ways. Sometimes His answers come in a sermon, sometimes in a book, sometimes in a thought, and sometimes in the words of a friend. Sometimes He leads us to just the right assistant. Sometimes He helps us know exactly the best decision possible. Sometimes our doctors prescribe just the right medication. Sometimes we find that parking space just when we need it most. God works in a multitude of ways. He is faithful. He loves me. He loves you. Forever.

Faith Endures

The autumn leaves are turning brown
while flowers shrivel to the ground.
Family members have passed on.
Their hugs and kisses are now gone.

Faith endures past what we know
like seeds alive grow under snow.
We find those we love once again.
They're not so far around the bend.

Dear Reader,

Please write to me at **rbbbadowski@hotmail.com**. I look forward to reading about your experiences as a caregiver.

God Bless You,
Veronica

My husband Bill and I live in the Northeast with our two cats, Misu and Silver Belle. Summers we camp near Portland, Maine where we spend many days visiting or relaxing at the seashore with our daughter Kelly, her husband Kurt, and our grandson John. Often, we vacation at Eufaula, Alabama where we rent a cabin on the beautiful Chattahoochee River. During this time, we take many interesting hikes with our son Keith and his wife Christi.

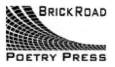

Our Mission

The mission of Brick Road Poetry Press is to publish and promote poetry that entertains, amuses, edifies, and surprises a wide audience of appreciative readers. We are not qualified to judge who deserves to be published, so we concentrate on publishing what we enjoy. Our preference is for poetry geared toward dramatizing the human experience in language rich with sensory image and metaphor, recognizing that poetry can be, at one and the same time, both familiar as the perspiration of daily labor and as outrageous as a carnival sideshow.

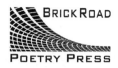

Also Available from Brick Road Poetry Press
www.brickroadpoetrypress.com

Dancing on the Rim by Clela Reed

Possible Crocodiles by Barry Marks

Pain Diary by Joseph D. Reich

Otherness by M. Ayodele Heath

Drunken Robins by David Oates

Damnatio Memoriae by Michael Meyerhofer

Lotus Buffet by Rupert Fike

The Melancholy MBA by Richard Donnelly

Two-Star General by Grey Held

Chosen by Toni Thomas

Etch and Blur by Jamie Thomas

Water-Rites by Ann E. Michael

Bad Behavior by Michael Steffen

Tracing the Lines by Susanna Lang

Rising to the Rim by Carol Tyx

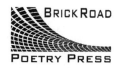

About the Prize

The Brick Road Poetry Prize, established in 2010, is awarded annually for the best book-length poetry manuscript. Entries are accepted August 1st through November 1st. The winner receives $1000 and publication. For details on our preferences and the complete submission guidelines, please visit our website at www.brickroadpoetrypress.com.